Diabetes
Meals on the Run

Fast, Healthy Menus Using Convenience Foods

BETTY WEDMAN-ST. LOUIS, PH.D., R.D., L.D.

Contemporary Books

*Chicago New York San Francisco Lisbon London Madrid Mexico City
Milan New Delhi San Juan Seoul Singapore Sydney Toronto*

Library of Congress Cataloging-in-Publication Data

Wedman-St. Louis, Betty.
    Diabetes meals on the run : convenience food menus for people with
diabetes / Betty Wedman-St. Louis.
        p.   cm.
    Includes bibliographical references and index.
    ISBN 0-8092-9788-4 (alk. paper)
    1. Diabetes—Diet therapy—Recipes. 2. Convenience foods. I. Title.

RC662 .W3628   2002
616.4'620654—dc21   2002019006

Contemporary Books

A Division of The *McGraw·Hill* Companies

1 2 3 4 5 6 7 8 9 0   DOC/DOC   1 0 9 8 7 6 5 4 3 2

ISBN 0-8092-9788-4

This book was set in Minion by Robert S. Tinnon Design
Printed and bound by R. R. Donnelley—Crawfordsville

Cover design by Jennifer Locke
Cover photo by Chris Everard/Getty Images
Interior design by Robert S. Tinnon

McGraw-Hill books are available at special quantity discounts to use as premiums and
sales promotions, or for use in corporate training programs. For more information,
please write to the Director of Special Sales, Professional Publishing, McGraw-Hill,
Two Penn Plaza, New York, NY 10121-2298. Or contact your local bookstore.

This book is printed on acid-free paper.

To Susan M. Busekrus, whose secretarial and office management expertise have provided me the opportunity to publish the many books and teaching aids for people with diabetes.

Contents

Preface

*D*iabetes is a chronic disease you learn to live with 365 days a year, 24 hours a day. It is no secret that you may not always stick to your medication, exercise, and meal planning regime. Blood glucose monitoring may not be done always as scheduled. The important key to good diabetes management is being realistic about how you want to control your blood glucose.

Guilt is a common reaction in diabetes. Education and evaluation can help overcome some of these emotional burdens, especially when it comes to meal planning issues. Each person needs to learn what is happening within his or her body and how to modify the consequences through proper meal planning, exercise, and medication (if needed).

The emotional aspects of food, however, can make meal planning issues seem overwhelming. The meal plan needs to be modified to meet an individual lifestyle. Forget about the word *cheating* and think of treats as *liberties* instead. How frequent and how often one eats treats is an individual decision. Remember that a planned liberty produces less guilt than an unplanned one.

The ideal diet for a person with diabetes remains to be determined. Most recommendations are for a low-fat, high-carbohydrate diet. The premise for this recommendation is based on reducing the risk of coronary heart disease. Others believe that a low-fat diet may promote weight reduction. The use of high-carbohydrate diets in people with diabetes who are overweight is coming under critical review. High-carbohydrate diets in this population can increase hyperglycemia, raise triglycerides, and lower high-density lipoproteins. In these cases, use of unsaturated fats (olive oil, avocado, etc.) is recommended instead of high carbohydrates.

As insulin reserves decline, individuals with diabetes will need to modify their diets to a lower carbohydrate regime. Therefore, the ideal diet for each person depends on his or her body weight and the stage of progression of beta cell dysfunction.

Balanced and optimal nutrient intake is important. Today's lifestyles and eating habits can often result in less-than-ideal levels of all essential nutrients. In addition, medical science is recognizing that each person has biochemical individuality, or distinct nutritional needs. Eating on the run and using convenience meals may not provide all the nutrients required; therefore, a balanced vitamin and mineral supplement program is an excellent way to ensure that these needs are met.

Acknowledgments

I wish to thank the many excellent diabetes educators who told me they needed a book like *Diabetes Meals on the Run: Convenience Food Menus for People with Diabetes.* Eating habits have drastically changed since my first nutrition course more than 35 years ago. Gone are the days of sliced bread and frozen vegetables as the convenience foods found in the local supermarket. Today, abundant, frozen complete meals are fast replacing the shelf space once devoted to flour, sugar, and shortening.

Times have also changed in the meal planning goals for people with diabetes. I wish to thank the many individuals who were open and honest enough to tell me how they *really* ate. It takes a lot of courage to ask a nutritionist how to fit a candy bar into a diabetic meal plan. After explaining how the American Diabetes Association (ADA) guidelines on sugar have changed over the years, a sample meal plan—like the one included in this book—was designed.

Yes, times have changed. My first menu and recipe book for people with diabetes included a chocolate chip cookie recipe that had about one-half teaspoon of sugar per cookie (far less than other homemade and store-bought varieties). The ADA would not allow me to include that recipe because the chocolate chips contained sugar and saturated fat. The current meal planning guidelines for people with diabetes focus more on total carbohydrates and limiting saturated fat in the diet. The ADA has finally come to accept that people are going to eat chocolate chip cookies regardless of whether they have diabetes or not. So, thanks to the new philosophy at the ADA, convenience foods with sugar are acceptable in the daily menu.

Introduction

*T*aste and convenience are the buzzwords for eating in this new millennium. The lack of time to prepare meals at home in the traditional manner has led to a wide array of prepared foods. Today, many meal planners don't start making dinner decisions before 4:00 P.M. Recent research on consumer trends indicates that almost 80 percent of adults eat at 6:00 P.M. or later, which increases the need for meals in a minute.

To challenge tradition even more, cleanup is what consumers dread the most about meal preparation. Convenience meals reduce dishes and minimize kitchen chores.

What You Eat Is Important

Eating is an important personal experience that holds cultural, social, and emotional meaning. What we eat, and how much, can be related to our values in life. The meaning of food is special to each person because eating is an event in which each person is in charge of his or her own choices.

Behavior change related to food choices in diabetes management is an ongoing process. Commitment to making dietary changes can vary from month to month and year to year. One of the first behavior changes in diabetes management is making a positive emotional adjustment to balancing food intake, exercise, and medication needs. Another step in behavior modification for blood glucose control is accepting responsibility for whatever choices are made in food intake, exercise regime, and medication adjustments.

Many people with diabetes are advised to follow a recommended meal plan. This meal planning guide is designed to provide less stress in the kitchen by choosing convenience foods that please the palate and allow guilt-free blood glucose management. Most meal plans assume home-cooked meals. A 1996 Roper Starch Worldwide study found that 86 percent of households purchase convenience entrées and that takeout meals doubled in the 1990s. *Diabetes Meals on the Run* provides meal plans for that changing American culture.

Dinner = Poured from a Bag

In 1980, no one would have believed that "home cooked" would mean poured from a plastic bag into a skillet. Supermarkets continue to increase their freezer sections while the food industry develops an increasing array of ultrafast meal items. The frozen-food aisles will undoubtedly become the most important section in the supermarket in the near future.

In 1990, consumers picked up frozen ingredients for mixing together a meal that took an hour or more to prepare. Today, a pair of scissors opens pouches and boxes that take on a homemade appeal because they are heated in the kitchen. A mere 10 to 15 minutes is all that many consumers allow for dinner preparation.

Frozen meal sales in the United States topped $1.3 billion in 1998, according to the July 1999 issue of *Food Processing*, yet there seems to be a growing demand for fresh packaged convenience foods from delis and refrigerated cases in the supermarket. The "3-day rule" on fresh convenience foods will continue to haunt retailers as conscientious consumers read the label and request more fresh convenience foods with a shelf life of less than 3 days!

TBC-TTG

The typical consumer who fills up the shopping cart with convenience items is TBC-TTG: Too Busy to Cook, Too Tired to Go out. Those who fall into this category include working couples with double incomes, frequently with children. Over 25 percent of these consumers believe that weekday dinners are not worth the effort to spend much time in the kitchen, according to Zara Champion in the May/June 1999 issue of *The World of Ingredients.*

During the work week, 72 percent of consumers in a supermarket study say they spend between 16 and 45 minutes preparing dinner. Therefore, the meals and recipes in *Diabetes Meals on the Run* have been designed with that in mind. On weekends, consumers usually spend more time on food preparation. Thirty-six percent of consumers in that same study reported spending at least 45 minutes preparing dinner during the weekend. This book features menus and recipes for quick meals for weekends and convenience menus using prepared foods for weekday meals.

Barbecue

Americans may not like to cook, but they do like to barbecue. More than 13 million owned grills in 1998. Barbecue-related food products have robust sales along with ready-to-eat or frozen meal accompaniments. Cooking in the home and grilling are fast becoming a "heat from the package" art. Recipes such as Lemon-Dill Chicken, Orange Herbed Pork Tenderloin, and Grilled Shrimp Cocktail are great for the grill.

Streamlining Your Dining

Americans are always in a hurry, with a pace of living approaching warp speed. *Diabetes Meals on the Run* is designed to help the stressed-out consumer who is looking for easy food preparation with time-saving options. You could say that "minute rice" isn't fast enough any more because it takes time to plan, purchase, and cook. Chapter 4, "Menus for Quick Meals," and Chapter 5, "Recipes for Quick Meals," feature 14 days of menus, and recipes having only four or five ingredients. Many people believe that home-prepared foods are more nutritious, and they are willing to spend the few extra minutes for that improved quality.

On the other hand, those wanting to spend the least amount of time in the kitchen will find Chapter 6, "Menus Featuring Prepared Foods," just what they are looking for. Fourteen days of convenience food meals have been designed so that breakfast, lunch, and dinner can be as easy as reading the directions on the prepared-food package. Tables of "Prepared-Food Comparisons" in Chapter 7 allow quick reference for selecting other brands or substituting a similar product.

Diabetes Meals on the Run is designed to be a handy guide to keep with you at all times. Shopping in the supermarket is easier with this book of comparisons. The menus allow for easy reference on how quickly a meal can be prepared with minimum ingredients.

Given today's time pressure, this book can provide the nutritional guidelines to help keep you on track in diet management of diabetes. Gone are the days when mom made breakfast for the family every day and the family sat down for dinner every night. It's a different pace than in the 1950s and 1960s. Today, breakfast is "catch as you can," lunch is a meal replacement bar, and dinner is frequently eaten "out of a box" to minimize planning and cleanup.

Chapter 1
Diabetes Meal Planning Basics

*W*hen you have diabetes, you need to decide when to eat, what to eat, and how much to eat on a more consistent basis than someone who doesn't have diabetes.

Healthy meals include foods with protein, carbohydrate, and fat for good blood glucose control. Another goal in diabetes meal planning is keeping blood lipids (cholesterol and triglycerides) in normal range to reduce the risk of heart disease. Weight management is a key factor in diabetes meal planning because overeating leads to extra calories that are stored as fat.

Carbohydrate Counting

Some people with diabetes manage their blood glucose by *carbohydrate counting*. The key to determining how high and how quickly your blood glucose level goes up is based on the type and amount of food eaten. Carbohydrates in foods affect your blood glucose the most, so knowing how many carbohydrates are eaten can help you manage your blood glucose level better.

Carbohydrates are found in starchy foods and sugar. Sugar includes the sweeteners that are present in foods naturally and those added to foods. These foods include breads, cereals, crackers, cookies, pasta, rice, potatoes, fruits, vegetables, milk, honey, syrup, brown sugar, white sugar, and molasses.

Eating the same amount of carbohydrates (plus or minus 5 to 10 grams) at each meal and snack is important in fine-tuning blood glucose management. Consistency in serving size and carbohydrate levels makes postmeal blood glucose levels easier to predict. You and a dietitian or nutritionist need to decide how much carbohydrate to eat at each meal. The total amount of carbohydrates in a daily menu is spaced throughout the day to make it easier to maintain a normal blood glucose level.

A small bowl of cereal one morning for breakfast will have fewer carbohydrates than a large bowl the next day. Eating one slice of toast one morning and two slices the next day does not allow for good blood glucose management.

Food labels can be useful in carbohydrate counting. One serving may equal the serving size listed in the food exchange list (see Appendix) and may have a similar carbohydrate amount. An example is the apple juice nutrition label in Figure 1.1.

The apple juice label indicates that the serving size of ½ cup = 15 grams carbohydrate. The food exchange list also identifies apple juice (½ cup) as having 15 grams carbohydrate.

When it comes to reading the food labels on prepared convenience foods, the carbohydrate levels will probably not match anything in the food exchange lists. You need to calculate your total carbohydrates in a specific

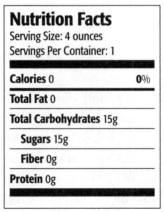

Figure 1.1 Apple Juice Label

meal and choose foods that fit within the range established by your dietitian or nutritionist.

An example is a noon meal with two slices of bread (two starch exchanges) × 15 grams carbohydrate = 30 grams. One fruit × 15 grams and 1 milk × 12 grams brings your noon meal total to 57 grams. Your prepared-food choices can include 55 to 60 grams of carbohydrates.

Protein and Fat

Protein and fat levels in foods may not raise your blood glucose level as high as carbohydrates, but they are important to consider in the meal plan. The quantity and type of fat are very important in weight management and controlling diabetes complications of coronary heart disease. Increasing the amount of unsaturated fats (vegetable oils, avocado, nuts, fish) instead of saturated fats from fried foods and trans fats in prepared desserts is recommended.

Calorie Counting

Calorie counting is generally used in weight-loss programs for those with non-insulin-dependent diabetes. This approach enables you to control calories to achieve a 1 to 2 pound per week weight loss. The best way to cut calories is to reduce portion sizes. Eating too much of a good food leads to weight gain, just like eating too much of an unhealthy food.

Although calorie counting is effective for some people with diabetes, it does not take into account a food's glycemic effect or carbohydrate content. No medication adjustment protocols are available for this approach, so support from the health care team is necessary. Losing weight slowly may not give instant gratification but chances are you may keep it off longer.

Glycemic Index

The use of the glycemic index in diabetes meal planning is divided by geographic boundaries. Research resulting in the glycemic index has increased our understanding of how foods are digested in the body. Australia, New Zealand, Canada, the United Kingdom, and France have adopted the glycemic index for diabetic meal planning. The American Diabetes Association prefers the carbohydrate counting method based on research defining carbohydrates as the major determinant for postmeal blood glucose response.

The glycemic index as reported in *Diabetes Care* grouped single foods by blood glucose response curves. A 50-gram portion (about 2 ounces) of available carbohydrate was fed to healthy volunteers. Blood glucose levels were drawn from 2 to 4 hours later to see how much each food raised blood glucose responses. Some testing was also done on individuals with diabetes.

It turned out that low glycemic index foods were not always high complex carbohydrate (starchy) foods. Sugary foods like candy bars (i.e., Mars bar) were not a high glycemic index food. Bread, breakfast cereals, and potatoes were rated higher on the glycemic scale than bananas, raisins, and sucrose. (See chart on page 9.)

The glycemic index research challenged the traditional belief that sugars (natural and added) would be rapidly absorbed and would raise blood glucose levels more than starches. This finding eventually led to the "liberalization" of using sugar in recipes and food products for diabetics.

Here are results of glycemic index research: Glucose sweetener raised blood glucose levels 100 percent. Corn flakes and instant mashed potatoes raised blood glucose level more than sucrose (table sugar) or potato chips. Ice cream had a lower glycemic effect than spaghetti or orange juice. No wonder this type of research has resulted in a new look at diabetes meal planning. Review these results with your diabetes educator to help you find the diet approach that will work best for you.

Glycemic Index of Selected Foods*

100%
Glucose

80%–90%
Corn flakes
Carrots[†]
Parsnips[†]
Potatoes (instant mashed)
Maltose
Honey

70%–79%
Bread (whole meal)
Millet
Rice (white)
Broad beans (fresh)[‡]
Potato (new)

60%–69%
Bread (white)
Rice (brown)
Muesli
Shredded Wheat
Water biscuits
Beetroot[†]
Bananas
Raisins
Mars bar

50%–59%
Buckwheat
Spaghetti (white)
Sweet corn
All-Bran
Digestive biscuits
Oatmeal biscuits

Peas (frozen)
Yam
Sucrose
Potato chips

40%–49%
Spaghetti (whole meal)
Porridge oats
Potato (sweet)
Beans (canned navy)
Peas (dried)
Oranges
Orange juice

30%–39%
Butter beans
Haricot beans
Blackeye peas
Chickpeas
Apples (Golden Delicious)
Ice cream
Milk (skim)
Milk (whole)
Yogurt
Tomato soup

20%–29%
Kidney beans
Lentils
Fructose

10%–19%
Soya beans
Soya beans (canned)
Peanuts

* Data from normal individuals.

† Table reproduced with permission from the American Diabetes Association, Inc., from D. J. A. Jenkins, Lente carbohydrate: A newer approach to the dietary management of diabetes. *Diabetes Care* 5 (1982): 634.

‡ 25-gram carbohydrate portions tested.

Chapter 2
Food Safety

Supermarkets today cater to the time-harried consumer as well as the more astute individual who realizes that food safety is important. Prepared ready-to-eat foods present many challenges to ensure that microbiological quality and safety are not compromised.

Refrigerated foods have a limited shelf life compared with frozen prepared foods. Microorganisms can grow even during refrigerated storage. Bacteria, yeasts, and molds reduce the flavor and texture of the food in addition to producing toxins that can cause food-borne illnesses.

Good manufacturing practices, sanitation, and employee hygiene serve as control methods to minimize microbial contamination of prepared foods. Manufacturers, however, recognize the potential for temperature abuse during distribution or storage of foods. Keeping prepared foods refrigerated or frozen is necessary to ensure optimum taste and to minimize the possibility of food-borne illness. Foods should be placed at proper storage temperatures within 30 minutes of purchase to retain freshness and quality. Refrigerated or frozen meals taken to work or school should be kept cold until ready to eat. Defrosting at room temperature increases the risk of bacteria contamination.

Salad Bars

According to most health inspectors, salad bars are the riskiest factor in eating. There are not enough inspectors to oversee supermarkets, delis, and restaurant salad bars to keep food safety under control. Because food loaded with harmful bacteria is seldom life threatening, many people are unaware of the health hazards.

The chances of getting food from a salad bar that is not clean and fresh are greater than most consumers believe. People pick up pieces of fruit with their fingers. Another individual "tastes" the tuna salad by running a finger along the edge of the serving container. Who knows where those fingers have been before sampling foods at the salad bar.

There are no specifications as to how long a food can stay on a salad bar or in a deli display case. Some establishments add fresh product on top of leftovers. Others leave containers of salad bar foods sitting at room temperature for hours until all the containers have been refilled, allowing significant breeding time for bacteria toxins that thrive at 60° to 100°F.

High bacteria counts in food can cause gastrointestinal problems, especially among people whose immune systems are compromised. Most digestive distress is never reported because it is so difficult to trace. Establishments are subject to a fine if high bacteria counts are found by health inspectors. Food service workers, however, frequently lack the motivation and training for keeping salad bars microbiologically safe.

It's a good idea to pass up some foods on the salad bar such as cantaloupe and alfalfa sprouts. The bacterial contamination of alfalfa sprouts is very difficult to wash away, even after a thorough soaking. Melons with ridges on the outer skin are difficult to wash clean of surface bacteria, viruses, or toxins. Cantaloupes and other foods grown with sewage as a fertilizer may contain these microbiological contaminants. Be safe, not sorry, when selecting foods from the salad bar.

The table on pages 13 to 14 can help identify some of the foods that cause food-borne illnesses and the symptoms of such illnesses.

Food-Borne Bacteria, Viruses, and Toxins

Name	Possible Symptoms (from most to least common)	Foods That Have Caused Outbreaks	How Soon It Typically Strikes	How Soon It Typically Ends
Campylobacter (bacteria)	Diarrhea (can be bloody), fever, abdominal pain, nausea, headache, muscle pain	Chicken, raw milk	2–5 days	7–10 days
Clostridium botulinum (bacteria)	Marked fatigue; weakness; dizziness; double vision; difficulty speaking, swallowing, and breathing; abdominal distention	Home-canned foods, sausages, meat products, commercially canned vegetables, seafood products	18–36 hours	Get treatment immediately
Cyclospora (parasite)	Watery diarrhea, loss of appetite, weight loss, cramps, nausea, vomiting, muscle aches, low-grade fever, extreme fatigue	Raspberries, lettuce, basil	1 week	A few days to 30 days or more
E. coli (bacteria)	Severe abdominal pain, watery (then bloody) diarrhea, occasional vomiting	Ground beef, raw milk, lettuce, sprouts, unpasteurized juices	1–8 days	Get treatment immediately
Hepatitis A (virus)	Fever, malaise, nausea, loss of appetite, abdominal pain, jaundice	Shellfish, salads, cold cuts, sandwiches, fruits, vegetables, fruit juices, milk, milk products, infected food handlers	10–50 days	1–2 weeks

Continued overleaf

Food Borne Bacteria, Viruses, Toxins, *continued*

Name	Possible Symptoms (from most to least common)	Foods That Have Caused Outbreaks	How Soon It Typically Strikes	How Soon It Typically Ends
Listeria (bacteria)	Fever, chills, and other flulike symptoms; headache; nausea; vomiting; diarrhea; infections of the blood (septicemia); inflammation of the brain (encephalitis) or membranes of the brain or spinal cord (meningitis); spontaneous abortion or stillbirth	Hot dogs, deli meats, raw milk, cheeses (particularly soft-ripened cheeses like feta, Brie, Camembert, blue-veined, or Mexican-style "queso blanco"), raw and cooked poultry, raw meats, ice cream, raw vegetables, raw and smoked fish	A few days to 3 weeks	Get treatment immediately
Norwalk virus (virus)	Nausea, vomiting, diarrhea, abdominal pain, headache, low-grade fever	Shellfish, salads, infected food handlers	1–2 days	1–2½ days
Salmonella (bacteria)	Nausea, vomiting, abdominal cramps, diarrhea, fever, headache	Poultry, eggs, raw meats, milk and dairy products, fish, shrimp, sauces and salad dressings, cream-filled desserts and toppings, fresh produce (including sprouts)	6 hours to 2 days	1–2 days

Chapter 3
Reading the Nutrition Label

*L*abels offer one way of distinguishing between prepared food choices. Nutrition labels can make it easier to figure out what you are eating, but manufacturers can still manipulate the words and processes unless you are an informed consumer. Here are some terms you will find on the food labels.

Fat free: A food with 1 gram fat or less per serving. Beware of serving size statements; they may be very small compared with what you consider a serving size.

98% fat free: Indicates the amount of fat per food weight, not percent of calories from fat. If a food weighs 3 ounces (about 90 grams) and contains 2 grams of fat, it is "98% fat free." A cheese that states it is 85% fat free can still have 14 grams of fat per 3-ounce serving.

Light or **Lite:** A term used to identify foods that have one-third fewer calories than the traditional food. In some cases, it has been used to market foods with a 50 percent reduction in fat and/or sodium.

No cholesterol: A phrase that can be misleading because some foods using this term on the label never had any cholesterol in them originally. Cholesterol is found in animal products: dairy foods, meat, poultry, seafood, and eggs. Saturated fat content is of greater consequence when trying to manage blood lipid levels.

Low fat: 3 grams or less per serving.

Low sodium: Less than 140 milligrams per serving.

Very low sodium: Less than 35 milligrams per serving.

Low cholesterol: Less than 20 milligrams per serving.

Low calorie: Less than 40 calories per serving (frozen meals = less than 120 calories per 3.5 ounces).

No sugar added: Usually refers to foods made with sugar substitutes such as saccharine, sorbitol, maltatol, and aspartame. This term may also be seen on some food labels when fruit juice or fruit purées are the sweetening agent.

Sugar-free: Refers to less than 0.5 gram of sugar or sweetener per serving.

Reduced sugar: Means at least 25 percent less sugar per serving than the usual product.

Sodium-free: Less than 5 milligrams of sodium per serving.

High fiber: Means 5 grams or more of fiber is present per serving of the food.

Good source of fiber: Designates foods with 2.5 to 4.9 grams of fiber per serving.

More fiber or **Added fiber:** Identifies foods with at least 2.5 grams per serving *more* than the usual product.

Healthy: Can be used for foods that are low in fat and saturated fats; a serving cannot contain more than 480 milligrams of sodium or more than 60 milligrams of cholesterol.

Sugar

Two common misconceptions are that you should not eat sugar when trying to lose weight and that you should not have sugar at all if you have diabetes. *Sugar* is a term used to describe any simple carbohydrate found in natural foods as well as prepared foods. Even fruits and vegetables have sugar.

The major difference between the simple carbohydrates in pasta, potatoes, and white granulated sugar is that white granulated sugar does not contain the vitamins, minerals, and other nutrients found in natural foods. Hence, calories from granulated sugar are called "empty" calories.

Consumption of sugar has risen significantly since the 1980s, according to health professionals. There are about 10 teaspoons of added sugar in a 12-ounce soft drink and 7 teaspoons of sugar in 8 ounces of low-fat, fruit-flavored yogurt. A fast-food shake contains about 12 teaspoons of added sugar. Although there is no scientific data linking such high sugar intake to obesity, increased calories from sugar may easily be a contributing factor.

Sugar, though, plays an important role in eating. Our taste buds like sweetness. In fact, many of the fat-free prepared foods on the market are loaded with extra sugar to make up for the taste appeal lost from the reduced fat content.

Eating sugar as an ingredient in prepared foods—but not the predominate ingredient (unless it is a dessert)—is acceptable on a diabetic meal plan according to the American Diabetes Association.

Fat

Scratch the idea that a fat-free diet is a healthy diet. The truth is, there is no such thing as a fat-free diet unless it is synthetically made in a research kitchen. Fats are essential to health, and nature has made sure that a wide variety of foods are available to provide essential fatty acids for the transport of vitamins A, D, E, and K in the blood. Fats are also needed for many immune and endocrine functions, especially healthy hair and skin.

Butter Versus Margarine

Butter and margarine are the most frequently consumed sources of fat. The debate over which one to consume has the nutrition community divided. The presence of trans fatty acids in margarine resulting from hydrogenation of vegetable oils has tarnished the reputation of margarines as the spread of choice.

Rather than declaring one source better than another, it would be more prudent to recommend butter or margarine be used moderately and vegetable oils be selected for cooking and baking. Olive oil, avocado oil, and nut oils offer flavor and fatty acid benefits that take the sting out of reducing fat content in the diet.

Fat Comparisons

See if you think the nutrition information provided in the table on pages 19 to 21 warrants paying twice the price for special margarines such as Benecol and Take Control. Research studies have shown that the use of these spreads lowered low-density lipoprotein (LDL) cholesterol up to 14 percent—which is not a significant difference for the added cost. (An LDL cholesterol level of 321 lowered by 14 percent is 276; normal is 0–130.) Studies have not been done to show consistent lipid modifications. Reducing fat content in the diet could easily lower LDL cholesterol 10 to 15 percent without the use of special margarines.

This listing is not inclusive of every brand in the supermarket. It is a representation of the variety of products currently available. Nutrient values have been rounded to whole numbers for easier comparison.

Fat Comparisons

	Serving Size	Calories	Total Fat (g)	Saturated Fat (g)	Polyunsaturated Fat (g)	Monounsaturated Fat (g)	Cholesterol (mg)	Sodium (mg)
Margarines								
Benecol:								
Light	1 tbsp.	30	3	0	1	1	0	65
Regular	1 tbsp.	45	5	0	1	2	0	65
Blue Bonnet:								
Light stick	1 tbsp.	50	6	1	1	1	0	75
Stick	1 tbsp.	70	7	1	2	1	0	100
Tub	1 tbsp.	60	7	1	3	1	0	110
Fleischmann's:								
Low-fat margarine stick	1 tbsp.	50	6	1	2	1	0	75
Low-fat margarine tub	1 tbsp.	40	4	9	1	2	0	90
Margarine stick	1 tbsp.	100	11	2	3	3	0	115
Margarine unsalted stick	1 tbsp.	100	11	2	3	3	0	0
Original light tub	1 tbsp.	40	4	0	1	2	0	90
Original margarine tub	1 tbsp.	80	9	1	4	3	0	90
Original unsalted tub	1 tbsp.	80	9	1	4	2	0	0
I Can't Believe It's Not Butter:								
Easy squeeze	1 tbsp.	80	8	1	5	2	0	95
Light stick	1 tbsp.	50	6	1	1	1	0	90
Light tub	1 tbsp.	50	5	1	2	1	0	90
Nonfat spread tub	1 tbsp.	5	0	0	0	0	0	90

Continued overleaf

Fat Comparisons, continued

	Serving Size	Calories	Total Fat (g)	Saturated Fat (g)	Polyunsaturated Fat (g)	Monounsaturated Fat (g)	Cholesterol (mg)	Sodium (mg)
Regular stick	1 tbsp.	90	10	2	2	2	0	95
Regular tub	1 tbsp.	90	10	2	4	1	0	95
Land O'Lakes:								
Butter stick	1 tbsp.	100	11	8	2	0	30	85
Country Morning Blend light stick	1 tbsp.	50	6	3	1	1	10	110
Country Morning Blend margarine stick	1 tbsp.	100	11	2	3	3	0	90
Country Morning Blend margarine tub	1 tbsp.	100	11	2	4	3	0	80
Light butter stick	1 tbsp.	50	6	4	0	2	20	70
Light unsalted butter stick	1 tbsp.	50	6	4	0	2	20	0
Light whipped butter tub	1 tbsp.	35	3	2	0	1	10	45
Unsalted butter stick	1 tbsp.	100	11	8	2	0	30	0
Whipped butter tub	1 tbsp.	70	7	5	1	0	20	50
Parkay:								
Buttery spray	1 spray	0	0	0	0	0	0	5
Light stick	1 tbsp.	50	6	1	1	1	0	75
Stick	1 tbsp.	90	10	2	3	2	0	105
Tub	1 tbsp.	80	8	1	4	3	0	100
Promise:								
Buttery light stick	1 tbsp.	50	6	1	1	1	0	50
Buttery light tub	1 tbsp.	50	5	1	3	1	0	50
Regular stick	1 tbsp.	90	10	2	4	2	0	90

	Serving							
Regular tub	1 tbsp.	90	10	1	4	1	0	95
Ultra fat free	1 tbsp.	5	0	0	0	0	0	90
Ultra tub	1 tbsp.	30	3	0	1	2	0	55
Shedd's Spread:								
Country Crock stick	1 tbsp.	70	7	1	2	1	0	110
Country Crock tub	1 tbsp.	70	7	1	2	1	0	110
Take Control:								
Tub	1 tbsp.	50	6	0	2	2	<5	110
Oils								
Bertolli:								
Extra light olive	1 tbsp.	120	14	2	2	10	0	0
Olive	1 tbsp.	120	14	2	2	10	0	0
Crisco Vegetable	1 tbsp.	120	14	2	6	6	0	0
Hollywood:								
Canola	1 tbsp.	120	14	1	4	8	0	0
Peanut	1 tbsp.	120	14	2	5	7	0	0
Safflower	1 tbsp.	120	14	1	11	2	0	0
Loriva:								
California walnut	1 tbsp.	120	14	2	9	3	0	0
Rice bran	1 tbsp.	120	14	2	6	6	0	0
Toasted sesame	1 tbsp.	120	14	2	6	6	0	0
Mazola:								
Canola	1 tbsp.	120	14	1	4	8	0	0
Corn	1 tbsp.	120	14	2	8	3	0	0
Wesson Vegetable	1 tbsp.	120	14	2	8	3	0	0

Chapter 4
Menus for Quick Meals

Day 1

Breakfast

Bagel

Low-fat cream cheese

Orange juice

Lunch

Turkey Waldorf Salad on lettuce (page 64)

Crackers

Dinner

Flank Steak on Asian Slaw (page 63)

Baked sweet potato

Fresh fruit cup

Cookie

Day 2

Breakfast

Oatmeal Banana Smoothie (page 37)

Lunch

California Pizza (page 51)

Grapes

Dinner

Sherried Scallops (recipe on page 66)

Rice

Green beans

Mixed vegetable salad

Low-fat salad dressing

Raspberry Dip (page 79)

Day 3

Breakfast

Ready-to-eat cereal

Low-fat milk

Strawberries

Lunch

Chicken Salad with Mango (page 55)

Wild Rice Salad (page 73)

Oatmeal cookie

Dinner

Peppered Pork with Apricot Glaze (page 56)

Buttered noodles

Orange-glazed Carrots (page 72)

Spinach salad

Low-fat salad dressing

Day 4

Breakfast

Melon cubes

Peanut butter on toasted English muffin

Lunch

Moroccan Turkey Burgers (page 54)

Lettuce and tomato

Pear

Dinner

Shrimp Vermouth (page 65)

Rice

Peas and onions

Caesar salad

Chocolate Chip Bread Pudding (page 78)

Day 5

Breakfast

Cottage cheese on raisin toast

Grapefruit juice

Lunch

Zesty Refried Bean Dip (page 46)

Vegetables

(carrots, celery, green pepper strips, cucumber slices, broccoli florets)

Bread sticks

Dinner

Greek Chicken with Capers (page 45)

Garlic Fries (page 70)

Mixed vegetables

Blueberries

Day 6

Breakfast

Banana Soy Smoothie (page 38)

Lunch

Gazpacho (page 40)

Portobello Sandwich (page 42)

Sugar cookie

Dinner

Low-fat Tofu Alfredo (page 47)

Mixed vegetable salad

Low-fat salad dressing

Strawberries

Day 7

Breakfast

Instant oatmeal

Low-fat milk

Raisins

Lunch

Spaghetti Pie (page 50)

Mixed vegetable salad

Low-fat salad dressing

Peach

Dinner

Honey-glazed Salmon (page 68)

Buttered noodles

Broccoli spears

Granola Blueberry Crisp (page 81)

Day 8

Breakfast

Ready-to-eat cereal

Low-fat milk

Strawberries

Lunch

Mexican Tuna Salad (page 48)

Whole grain bread

Apple

Dinner

Swordfish with Fresh Tomatoes (page 49)

Roasted Potatoes with Pesto (page 71)

Spinach

Pound cake

Day 9

Breakfast

Breakfast Hot Dog (page 39)

Orange juice

Lunch

Grilled Shrimp Cocktail (page 67)

Croissant

Grapes

Dinner

Orange Herbed Pork Tenderloin (page 53)

French Potato Salad (page 74)

Mixed vegetable salad

Low-fat salad dressing

Kahlua Fudge Sauce (page 80)

Sponge cake squares

Day 10

Breakfast

Bagel

Low-fat cream cheese

Grapefruit juice

Lunch

Greek Chicken Salad (page 57)

Crackers

Orange wedges

Dinner

Ham and Broccoli Casserole (page 58)

Sliced tomato

Low-fat dressing

Fresh Peach Cake (page 77)

Day 11

Breakfast

Hard-cooked egg

Toasted English muffin

Butter or margarine

Melon cubes

Lunch

Spinach-Macaroni-Bean Salad (page 60)

Muffin

Apple

Dinner

Artichoke-Spinach Pizza (page 59)

Fresh fruit cup

Day 12

Breakfast

Instant oatmeal

Low-fat milk

Apricots

Lunch

Mediterranean Niçoise Salad (page 41)

Hard roll and butter or margarine

Melon wedge

Dinner

Spiced Turkey Breast with Peach Salsa (page 43)

Buttered noodles

Peas and onions

Angel food cake slice

Day 13

Breakfast
Toasted frozen waffle

Peanut butter

Orange juice

Lunch
Chicken Mandarin Orange Salad (page 62)

Bagel

Butter or margarine

Dinner
Lamb and Fig Kabobs (page 61)

Rice

Green beans

Tomato and cucumber salad

Low-fat salad dressing

Walnut Cake (page 76)

Day 14

Breakfast

Ready-to-eat cereal

Low-fat milk

Grapefruit juice

Lunch

Lemon-Dill Chicken (page 52)

Muffin

Mixed vegetable salad

Low-fat salad dressing

Grapes

Dinner

Salmon and Tomatoes En Parchment (page 69)

Noodles

Jalapeño Corn Muffins (page 75)

Asparagus

Fresh fruit in season

Chapter 5

Recipes for Quick Meals

Oatmeal Banana Smoothie

---

1 packet instant oatmeal
½ cup boiling water
1 medium banana, peeled
1 cup ice cubes

Blend cereal and boiling water together in blender at low speed for 1 minute. Add banana and ½ cup ice cubes. Blend on high speed until smooth, about 1 minute. Add remaining ice and blend until smooth. Serve immediately.

Makes 1 serving.

1 serving = 1 starch/bread + 2 fruit
Calories per serving = 166
Protein 2 g
Carbohydrates 28 g
Fat 0
Sodium 112 mg
Cholesterol 0

Banana Soy Smoothie

1 cup vanilla soy milk
1 small banana, peeled
4 to 5 toasted almonds
3 to 4 ice cubes

Blend all ingredients until smooth. Serve immediately.

Makes 1 serving.

1 serving = 1 lean meat or 1 low-fat milk + 2 fruit
Calories per serving = 159
Protein 8 g
Carbohydrates 35 g
Fat 5 g
Sodium 86 mg
Cholesterol 0

Breakfast Hot Dog

2 1-ounce turkey sausage breakfast links
1 hot dog roll
1 tablespoon shredded cheddar cheese

Cook sausage according to package directions. Toast hot dog roll in toaster oven. Put sausage links in roll. Top with cheese. Serve immediately.

Makes 1 serving.

1 serving = 3 medium-fat meat + 1 starch/bread
Calories per serving = 314
Protein 15 g
Carbohydrates 21 g
Fat 12 g
Sodium 342 mg
Cholesterol 97 mg

Gazpacho

1 small onion, chopped
1 green pepper, seeded and chopped
1 cucumber, peeled and seeded
1 to 2 cloves garlic, chopped
1 28-ounce can crushed tomatoes
Salt and pepper to taste

Combine onion, green pepper, cucumber, garlic, and tomatoes in blender. Puree until smooth. Season to taste with salt and pepper.
Chill until ready to serve.

Makes 4 servings.

1 serving = 2 vegetable
Calories per serving = 32
Protein 2 g
Carbohydrates 11 g
Fat 0
Sodium 51 mg
Cholesterol 0

Mediterranean Niçoise Salad

2 large lettuce leaves
1 3.5-ounce can water-packed tuna, drained
4 whole black olives
1 small ripe tomato, cut into chunks
1 pickling cucumber, peeled and sliced
2 tablespoons prepared low-fat Italian dressing

Line plate with washed lettuce leaves. Arrange tuna, olives, tomato, and cucumber on lettuce. Drizzle salad dressing over salad ingredients.

Makes 1 serving.

1 serving = 3 lean protein + 2 vegetable + 1 fat
Calories per serving = 241
Protein 24 g
Carbohydrates 12 g
Fat 4 g
Sodium 418 mg
Cholesterol 22 mg

Portobello Sandwich

1 teaspoon olive oil
1 cup sliced Portobello mushroom caps
1 slice sweet onion
2 slices sourdough bread
1-ounce slice provolone cheese

Heat olive oil in skillet over medium heat. Add mushrooms and onion.
Sauté about 5 minutes or until onion is tender. Cool.
Spread mushroom and onion mixture on 1 slice of bread. Top with cheese and
remaining slice of bread. Serve immediately.

Makes 1 serving.

1 serving = 2 medium-fat meat + 2 starch/grain
Calories per serving = 329
Protein 12 g
Carbohydrates 35 g
Fat 11 g
Sodium 192 mg
Cholesterol 22 mg

Spiced Turkey Breast with Peach Salsa

1 3- to 4-pound fresh turkey breast
½ teaspoon ground cinnamon
¼ teaspoon ground ginger
⅛ teaspoon ground cloves
Peach salsa (see page 44)

Place turkey breast in shallow roasting pan. Combine cinnamon, ginger, and
cloves in small bowl. Stir to blend. Rub spice mixture onto skin.
Bake in preheated 350°F oven 45 to 50 minutes. Test for doneness.

Makes 6 servings.

1 serving = 4 lean meat + ½ fruit
Calories per serving (with salsa) = 256
Protein 31 g
Carbohydrates 8 g
Fat 4 g
Sodium 87 mg
Cholesterol 106 mg

Peach Salsa

1 cup fresh or frozen peach slices
1 tablespoon chopped fresh parsley
¼ teaspoon ground cinnamon
2 tablespoons orange juice
½ tablespoon seeded and chopped jalapeño pepper (optional)

Combine all ingredients in food processor.
Process until blended. Chill until ready to serve.

Makes 1 cup or 4 servings.

1 serving (¼ cup) = ½ fruit
Calories per serving = 28
Protein 0
Carbohydrates 8 g
Fat 0
Sodium 2 mg
Cholesterol 0

Greek Chicken with Capers

2 4-ounce skinless, boneless chicken breast halves
½ teaspoon dried oregano
2 teaspoons olive oil
2 tablespoons capers
¼ cup (1 ounce) crumbled feta cheese

Sauté chicken breasts sprinkled with oregano in olive oil for 4 to 5 minutes on each side at medium heat. Cover; reduce heat to simmer for 5 to 10 minutes or until chicken is done. Add capers and cheese to pan. Stir until cheese makes sauce. Serve each chicken breast topped with caper and cheese sauce.

Makes 2 servings.

1 serving = 3 lean meat + 1 fat
Calories per serving = 222
Protein 25 g
Carbohydrates 3 g
Fat 8 g
Sodium 416 mg
Cholesterol 84 mg

Zesty Refried Bean Dip

1 small onion, chopped (about ¼ cup)
2 tablespoons prepared salsa
1 16-ounce can fat-free refried beans
1 ounce grated cheddar cheese (¼ cup)
Chopped fresh cilantro

Combine onion, salsa, and beans in food processor. Puree until smooth. Pour into microwave-proof bowl. Cook on high 2 minutes. Add cheese; stir till melted. Sprinkle on cilantro.

Makes 1½ cups.

1 serving (¼ cup) = 1 starch/bread
Calories per serving = 94
Protein 6 g
Carbohydrates 19 g
Fat 2 g
Sodium 319 mg
Cholesterol 29 mg

Low-fat Tofu Alfredo

4 ounces soft tofu
½ cup low-fat cottage cheese
2 tablespoons grated Parmesan cheese
1 small clove garlic
1½ cups cooked fettucini noodles
Chopped fresh parsley

Puree tofu, cottage cheese, Parmesan cheese, and garlic in food processor.
Pour into microwave-proof bowl. Cook on high in microwave 2 to 3 minutes
or until mixture bubbles. Pour over fettucini noodles.
Sprinkle with parsley just before serving.

Makes 2 servings.

1 serving = 4 lean meat + 1 starch/bread
Calories per serving = 297
Protein 31 g
Carbohydrates 28 g
Fat 6 g
Sodium 396 mg
Cholesterol 64 mg

Mexican Tuna Salad

1 6-ounce can water-packed tuna, drained
1 tablespoon reduced-fat mayonnaise
1 tablespoon prepared salsa
½ green pepper, seeded and chopped

Combine ingredients in bowl. Stir to mix. Use as salad or sandwich spread.

Makes 2 servings.

1 serving = 3 lean meat + 1 fat
Calories per serving = 191
Protein 20 g
Carbohydrates 4 g
Fat 4 g
Sodium 237 mg
Cholesterol 110 mg

Swordfish with Fresh Tomatoes

¾ pound swordfish steaks
2 teaspoons olive oil
1 ripe tomato, chopped
1 small clove garlic, minced
½ teaspoon dried thyme leaves *or*
1 teaspoon minced fresh thyme leaves

Place swordfish steaks and olive oil in skillet. Sauté on high heat 3 minutes.
Turn steaks and sauté until done, about 3 minutes.
Combine tomatoes, garlic, and thyme in bowl.
Spoon onto steaks when ready to serve.

Makes 2 servings.

1 serving = 4 lean meat + 1 vegetable
Calories per serving = 232
Protein 27 g
Carbohydrates 4 g
Fat 5 g
Sodium 87 mg
Cholesterol 116 mg

Spaghetti Pie

8 ounces spaghetti noodles, cooked and drained
1 egg
1 pound lean ground beef, cooked
2 cups prepared pasta sauce
8 ounces shredded mozzarella cheese

Toss together spaghetti noodles and egg. Press noodles into lightly oiled
9-inch pie pan to form crust. Mix ground beef and pasta sauce.
Spread mixture over noodle crust. Sprinkle with mozzarella cheese.
Bake in preheated 350°F oven 20 to 25 minutes or until thoroughly heated.
Let stand 5 minutes before cutting into wedges.

Makes 8 servings.

1 serving = 3 medium-fat meat + 1 starch/bread
Calories per serving = 334
Protein 26 g
Carbohydrates 23 g
Fat 7 g
Sodium 271 mg
Cholesterol 149 mg

California Pizza

1 prepared pizza crust
1 tablespoon olive oil
1 tablespoon minced fresh garlic
½ pound lean ham, sliced thin
½ pound provolone cheese, sliced thin

Drizzle pizza crust with olive oil. Sprinkle on garlic. Cut ham and cheese into strips and arrange on pizza crust. Bake in preheated 400°F oven 12 to 15 minutes or until cheese is melted.

Makes 4 servings.

Variations: MILD: Add ½ cup roasted red peppers, sliced into thin strips. SPICY: Add ¼ cup hot cherry peppers, sliced thinly.

1 serving = 2 starch/bread + 4 medium-fat meat
Calories per serving = 442
Protein 31 g
Carbohydrates 35 g
Fat 24 g
Sodium 716 mg
Cholesterol 99 mg

Lemon-Dill Chicken

2 4-ounce boneless, skinless chicken breasts
1 tablespoon olive oil
2 tablespoons lemon juice
1 tablespoon dried dill weed

Place chicken breasts in skillet with olive oil and lemon juice.
Sprinkle on dill weed. Sauté over medium heat 8 to 10 minutes
on each side or until tender.

Makes 2 servings.

1 serving = 3 lean meat + 1 fat
Calories per serving = 208
Protein 18 g
Carbohydrates 2 g
Fat 14 g
Sodium 151 mg
Cholesterol 106 mg

Orange Herbed Pork Tenderloin

12- to 16-ounce pork tenderloin
¼ cup orange marmalade
½ teaspoon dried thyme leaves
½ teaspoon ground rosemary
¼ teaspoon ground nutmeg

Place pork tenderloin on baking sheet. Combine rest of ingredients in bowl. Spread onto tenderloin. Bake in preheated 350°F oven 30 to 40 minutes or until meat thermometer registers 160°F. Slice and serve.

Makes 3 servings.

1 serving = 4 lean meat + 1 fruit
Calories per serving = 254
Protein 26 g
Carbohydrates 10 g
Fat 12 g
Sodium 198 mg
Cholesterol 129 mg

Moroccan Turkey Burgers

1 pound ground turkey
½ cup chopped onion
¼ cup pitted green olives, chopped
¼ cup raisins or currants
4 hamburger rolls, toasted

Combine ground turkey, onion, olives, and raisins in bowl. Mix well.
Divide into four equal portions. Shape each into 1-inch-thick patty.
Place in skillet over medium heat. Cook 6 minutes on each side
until no longer pink. Place burger on hamburger roll. Serve with catsup.

Makes 4 burgers.

1 serving = 3 lean meat + 2 starch/bread
Calories per serving = 391
Protein 26 g
Carbohydrates 41 g
Fat 18 g
Sodium 692 mg
Cholesterol 96 mg

Chicken Salad with Mango

2 4-ounce boneless, skinless chicken breasts
1 cup peeled and sliced mango (1 large)
½ cup thinly sliced green onions
2 tablespoons minced fresh ginger or ¼ teaspoon ground ginger
⅓ cup raspberry vinaigrette salad dressing
Salad greens

Grill or broil chicken breasts about 6 minutes on each side, or until done.
Cut chicken diagonally across grain into thin slices. Combine chicken,
mango, green onions, ginger, and salad dressing in mixing bowl.
Toss gently. Serve over salad greens.

Makes 2 servings.

1 serving = 3 lean meat + 1 fruit
Calories per serving = 222
Protein 26 g
Carbohydrates 7 g
Fat 4 g
Sodium 322 mg
Cholesterol 66 mg

Peppered Pork with Apricot Glaze

2 4-ounce boneless lean pork chops
1 teaspoon coarsely ground black pepper
2 tablespoons low-sugar apricot jam

Rub pork chops with pepper. Melt apricot jam in small microwave-proof
bowl on high for 25 seconds. Set aside. Cook chops over medium heat for
5 to 7 minutes on each side or until chops are no longer pink.
Drizzle apricot glaze over chops just before serving.

Makes 2 servings.

1 serving = 3 medium-fat meat
Calories per serving = 213
Protein 24 g
Carbohydrates 8 g
Fat 6 g
Sodium 63 mg
Cholesterol 80 mg

Greek Chicken Salad

3 cups chopped cooked chicken breast (about 12 ounces)
1 cup peeled, seeded, and diced cucumber
2 ounces (½ cup) crumbled feta cheese
¼ cup plain low-fat yogurt
½ cup low-fat mayonnaise
1 tablespoon dried oregano leaves

Combine all ingredients in mixing bowl. Toss well.
Refrigerate until ready to serve.

Makes 4 servings.

1 serving = 4 lean meat + 2 fat
Calories per serving = 305
Protein 26 g
Carbohydrates 7 g
Fat 12 g
Sodium 342 mg
Cholesterol 68 mg

Ham and Broccoli Casserole

2 cups cubed ham
1 10-ounce package frozen broccoli spears
Half of a 16-ounce jar cheese sauce
¼ teaspoon grated nutmeg
½ cup crumbled corn flakes

Place ham cubes and broccoli in microwave-proof dish.
Pour cheese sauce over ham and broccoli.
Sprinkle nutmeg and corn flakes over cheese sauce.
Microwave on high 2 minutes, just until bubbly.

Makes 3 servings.

1 serving = 3 medium-fat meat + ½ starch/bread + 1 fat + 1 vegetable
Calories per serving = 361
Protein 18 g
Carbohydrates 16 g
Fat 19 g
Sodium 407 mg
Cholesterol 114 mg

Artichoke-Spinach Pizza

1 10-ounce pizza crust
⅓ cup prepared feta cheese salad dressing
1 10-ounce package frozen, chopped spinach, thawed and drained
1 14-ounce can quartered artichoke hearts, drained
4 ounces grated provolone cheese *or*
shredded part-skim mozzarella cheese

Place pizza crust on baking sheet. Spread feta cheese salad dressing over crust. Top with spinach and artichoke hearts. Sprinkle on cheese. Bake in preheated 450°F oven 10 to 15 minutes or until cheese melts.

Makes 8 servings.

1 serving = 1 medium-fat protein + 1 starch/bread + 2 vegetable + 1 fat
Calories per serving = 248
Protein 12 g
Carbohydrates 28 g
Fat 14 g
Sodium 386 mg
Cholesterol 57 mg

Spinach-Macaroni-Bean Salad

2 cups chopped fresh spinach
2 cups cooked elbow macaroni (about 4 ounces uncooked)
¼ cup canned black beans, drained
1 cup chopped tomato
½ cup low-fat ranch salad dressing

Toss all ingredients together in mixing bowl. Chill until ready to serve.

Makes 2 servings.

(Ingredients can be heated in skillet over medium heat until hot,
about 3 minutes, for alternative vegetarian choice.)

1 serving = 1 lean meat + 2 starch/bread + 2 vegetable + 2 fat
Calories per serving = 342
Protein 8 g
Carbohydrates 39 g
Fat 12 g
Sodium 382 mg
Cholesterol 5 mg

Lamb and Fig Kabobs

2 pounds lean lamb chops
6 to 8 small cloves garlic, peeled
8 dried figs
¼ cup mint jelly
1 tablespoon olive oil

Trim fat and bone from lamb chops. Cut into bite-sized lamb cubes.
Thread skewers with lamb cubes, garlic cloves, and dried figs.
Place on broiler pan. Combine mint jelly and olive oil in microwave-proof bowl.
Heat 30 seconds on high to melt jelly. Baste lamb kabobs with jelly mixture.
Broil or grill until desired doneness.
Baste periodically with mint jelly mixture. Serve over rice.

Makes 2 servings.

1 serving = 3 medium-fat meat + 1 fruit
Calories per serving = 274
Protein 20 g
Carbohydrates 14 g
Fat 17 g
Sodium 162 mg
Cholesterol 97 mg

Chicken Mandarin Orange Salad

2 cups cooked chicken, cut into strips (1 pound boneless chicken breasts)
½ red sweet pepper, chopped
4 cups fresh salad greens
1 8-ounce can juice-packed mandarin oranges, drained
½ cup prepared raspberry vinaigrette dressing

Combine all ingredients in mixing bowl.
Toss gently. Serve chilled.

Makes 4 servings.

1 serving = 3 lean meat + 1 vegetable + 1 fruit

Calories per serving = 267
Protein 19 g
Carbohydrates 18 g
Fat 9 g
Sodium 174 mg
Cholesterol 89 mg

Flank Steak on Asian Slaw

1 to 1½ pounds beef flank steak
¼ cup low-fat French salad dressing
3 cups prepared cole slaw mixture (shredded cabbage and carrots)
2 scallions, thinly sliced, or 4 green onions
2 teaspoons sesame oil
1 tablespoon vegetable oil

Place flank steak on broiler pan and coat with French salad dressing.
Let stand while preparing slaw. Combine slaw mixture, scallions,
sesame oil, and vegetable oil in skillet. Sauté over medium heat just
until cabbage, carrots, and scallions are tender. Remove from heat.
Broil or grill flank steak until it reaches desired doneness,
about 8 minutes per side (medium doneness).
Stir slaw mixture and mound onto plate.
Slice steak thinly on bias and
drape slices over slaw.

Makes 4 servings.

1 serving = 3 medium-fat meat + 2 fat + 1 vegetable
Calories per serving = 337
Protein 24 g
Carbohydrates 8 g
Fat 23 g
Sodium 319 mg
Cholesterol 118 mg

Turkey Waldorf Salad

2 red-skinned apples
½ pound roast turkey, sliced ¼ inch thick
1 stalk celery (about 1 cup), chopped
¼ cup chopped walnuts
½ cup low-fat mayonnaise

Core apples and chop. Cut turkey into bite-sized pieces.
Mix with remaining ingredients in bowl.
Chill until ready to serve.

Makes 2 servings.

1 serving = 4 lean meat + 1 fruit + 2 fat
Calories per serving = 367
Protein 31 g
Carbohydrates 14 g
Fat 13 g
Sodium 308 mg
Cholesterol 111 mg

Shrimp Vermouth

1 tablespoon olive oil
½ cup minced shallots or onion
1 pound large fresh shrimp, peeled and deveined with tails left on
½ cup dry vermouth or white grape juice
¼ teaspoon hot sauce

Heat oil in skillet over medium heat. Add rest of ingredients.
Sauté 2 to 3 minutes until shrimp turn pink, stirring occasionally.
Serve over rice or noodles. Extra vermouth or hot sauce
may be added for individual taste.

Makes 3 servings.

1 serving = 3 lean meat + 1 fat
Calories per serving = 201
Protein 22 g
Carbohydrates 5 g
Fat 5 g
Sodium 211 mg
Cholesterol 118 mg

Sherried Scallops

1 tablespoon olive oil
1 pound bay or sea scallops
½ cup chopped onion
1 large clove garlic, minced
¼ cup dry sherry
1 14.5-ounce can whole tomatoes

Heat olive oil in skillet over medium heat. Add scallops and sauté 2 minutes.
Add onion, garlic, and sherry. Sauté 2 minutes or until onions are tender.
Add tomatoes; cook 2 minutes to heat thoroughly before serving.

Makes 4 servings.

1 serving = 3 lean meat + 1 vegetable
Calories per serving = 182
Protein 23 g
Carbohydrates 16 g
Fat 5 g
Sodium 372 mg
Cholesterol 83 mg

Grilled Shrimp Cocktail

16 to 20 large shrimp, peeled and deveined with tails left on
¼ cup creamy low-fat Italian dressing
¼ cup mayonnaise
1 clove garlic, minced
1 tablespoon lemon juice

Marinate shrimp in Italian dressing 15 to 20 minutes.
Thread onto two skewers. Broil 4 inches from heat for 3 minutes per side.
Brush with any leftover dressing.
Meanwhile, combine rest of ingredients in small bowl. Blend together well.
Serve shrimp skewers with lemon garlic mayonnaise for dipping.

Makes 2 servings.

1 serving = 3 lean meat + 2 fat
Calories per serving = 268
Protein 16 g
Carbohydrates 4 g
Fat 11 g
Sodium 329 mg
Cholesterol 178 mg

Honey-glazed Salmon

2 6-ounce salmon fillets
1 tablespoon honey
1 teaspoon Dijon mustard
½ teaspoon dried thyme leaves

Place salmon fillets on baking sheet or broiler pan.
Combine rest of ingredients in bowl.
Spoon mixture over skinless side of salmon.
Broil 5 to 6 minutes on each side or until fish flakes with fork.

Makes 2 servings.

1 serving = 4 lean meat
Calories per serving = 197
Protein 33 g
Carbohydrates 12 g
Fat 14 g
Sodium 310 mg
Cholesterol 110 mg

Salmon and Tomatoes En Parchment

12 to 16 ounces fresh salmon fillet, cut into two pieces
1 tablespoon olive oil
6 to 8 cherry tomatoes, cut in half
½ teaspoon dried basil leaves *or*
1 teaspoon fresh chopped basil leaves

Cut parchment (foil can be substituted) to fit each fillet of salmon.
Place fillet in center of parchment. Drizzle olive oil over fillets.
Add tomato pieces and basil leaves. Enclose fillets in parchment
by rolling top and sides. Place each packet on baking sheet.
Bake in preheated 400°F oven 12 to 15 minutes.
Open one packet and test fish for flakiness.
If not done, return to oven for 5 more minutes. Serve in parchment.

Makes 2 servings.

1 serving = 4 lean meat + 1 vegetable + 1 fat
Calories per serving = 271
Protein 33 g
Carbohydrates 3 g
Fat 16 g
Sodium 199 mg
Cholesterol 167 mg

Garlic Fries

¼ cup olive oil
¼ cup vegetable oil
1 pound frozen french fries
¼ cup minced garlic
¼ teaspoon salt

Combine oils in large skillet. Heat until hot. Add french fries.
Cook, stirring occasionally, until browned, about 3 to 4 minutes.
Drain on paper towel. Mix garlic and salt in small bowl.
Sprinkle over fries. Toss to coat. Serve hot.

Makes 2 servings.

1 serving = 1 starch/bread + 1 fat
Calories per serving = 171
Protein 2 g
Carbohydrates 18 g
Fat 8 g
Sodium 374 mg
Cholesterol 0

Roasted Potatoes with Pesto

2 cups frozen french fries
½ small cucumber, peeled and seeded
½ cup fresh parsley sprigs
2 tablespoons creamy Italian salad dressing
1 teaspoon dried basil leaves *or*
¼ cup fresh basil leaves

Bake french fries in 425°F oven 20 to 25 minutes.
Meanwhile, prepare pesto by combining remaining ingredients
in food processor. Puree until smooth. Combine french fries and pesto.
Toss to coat fries. Serve immediately.

Makes 2 servings.

1 serving = 1 starch/bread + 1 fat
Calories per serving = 147
Protein 2 g
Carbohydrates 23 g
Fat 7 g
Sodium 97 mg
Cholesterol 5 mg

Orange-glazed Carrots

4 to 5 medium carrots
1 red sweet pepper, diced
1 small onion, chopped fine
2 tablespoons low-sugar orange marmalade
Salt to taste

Peel and slice carrots into ½-inch-thick circles.
Steam carrots, red sweet pepper, and onion until tender,
about 5 to 7 minutes. Place in bowl.
Add orange marmalade and mix gently. Salt to taste.
Serve immediately.

Makes 2 servings.

1 serving = 2 vegetable
Calories per serving = 72
Protein 2 g
Carbohydrates 16 g
Fat 0
Sodium 28 mg (no salt added)

Cholesterol 0

Wild Rice Salad

½ cup uncooked wild rice
½ cup sliced fresh mushrooms
¼ cup chopped green onions
¼ cup low-fat ranch salad dressing
¼ cup toasted slivered almonds

Cook rice according to package directions. Drain and cool.
Combine rice, mushrooms, green onions, and salad dressing in bowl.
Toss gently. Chill until ready to serve.
Sprinkle on almonds just before serving.

Makes 2 servings.

1 serving = 1 starch/bread + 2 fat + 1 vegetable
Calories per serving = 189
Protein 3 g
Carbohydrates 24 g
Fat 11 g
Sodium 264 mg
Cholesterol 4 mg

French Potato Salad

1 pound potatoes
3 tablespoons white wine or white grape juice
½ teaspoon Dijon mustard
¼ teaspoon salt
2 tablespoons olive oil
Finely chopped green onion

Scrub potatoes and cut into bite-sized chunks.
Drop into boiling salted water. Boil 10 to 15 minutes or until potatoes
are fork tender. Drain off water. Cool potatoes in shallow serving dish.
Pour rest of ingredients over potatoes. Toss gently to blend.
Sprinkle with green onion before serving.

Makes 2 servings.

1 serving = 1 starch/bread + 2 fats
Calories per serving = 203
Protein 2 g
Carbohydrates 23 g
Fat 11 g
Sodium 282 mg
Cholesterol 0

Jalapeño Corn Muffins

1 7-ounce corn muffin mix
1 egg
2 tablespoons vegetable oil
2 jalapeño peppers, seeded and chopped fine

Pour muffin mix into bowl. Add water per package directions.
Stir in remaining ingredients. Pour batter into muffin cups.
Bake according to package directions.

Makes 6 servings.

1 serving = 1 starch/bread + 1 fat
Calories per serving = 119
Protein 2 g
Carbohydrates 17 g
Fat 6 g
Sodium 194 mg
Cholesterol 57 mg

Walnut Cake

1 18.25-ounce yellow cake mix
3 eggs
4 ounces walnuts
2 tablespoons rum *or*
1 teaspoon rum extract
1 tablespoon zest of orange (grated orange rind)

Prepare cake mix according to package directions using 3 eggs.
Place walnuts in food processor. Grind until fine, but not powdered.
Add to cake mixture. Stir in rum and zest of orange.
Pour batter into greased and floured 8-inch springform or
bundt cake pan. Bake in preheated 350°F oven 40 to 45 minutes
or until center of cake is dry when tested with toothpick.
Remove from pan. Cool.

Makes 12 servings.

1 serving = 1 starch/bread + 1 fruit + 2 fat

Calories per serving = 267
Protein 4 g
Carbohydrates 31 g
Fat 12 g
Sodium 347 mg
Cholesterol 69 mg

Fresh Peach Cake

2 cups coarsely chopped fresh or frozen peaches
2 tablespoons chopped pecans
1 tablespoon butter or margarine
1 18.25-ounce yellow cake mix
3 eggs
1 teaspoon ground cinnamon

Place peaches and pecans in bottom of oiled 8-inch-square baking pan.
Melt butter in microwave and drizzle over peaches.
Prepare cake mix according to package directions, using 3 eggs and
adding cinnamon to batter. Spoon batter over peach slices.
Bake in preheated 375°F oven 30 to 40 minutes or until golden brown.
Invert pan. Cool 5 minutes before removing. Serve warm or cold.

Makes 6 servings.

1 serving = 1 starch/bread + 1 fruit + 2 fat
Calories per serving = 257
Protein 3 g
Carbohydrates 29 g
Fat 13 g
Sodium 149 mg
Cholesterol 41 mg

Chocolate Chip Bread Pudding

8 chocolate chip cookies, broken into 1-inch pieces
1 slice bread, cut into small cubes
1 cup low-fat milk
2 eggs

Combine cookies and bread in greased 1-quart casserole.
Beat milk and eggs together. Pour over cookies and bread.
Bake in preheated 350°F oven 25 to 30 minutes.
Test for doneness by inserting knife into center.
When it comes out clean, remove from oven.
Let cool 5 to 10 minutes. Serve warm.

Makes 4 servings.

1 serving = 1 starch/bread + 1 fruit + 1 fat
Calories per serving = 203
Protein 5 g
Carbohydrates 32 g
Fat 8 g
Sodium 210 mg
Cholesterol 56 mg

Raspberry Dip

1 cup low-fat cottage cheese
1 cup frozen raspberries, thawed
2 tablespoons orange juice
Vanilla wafers

Blend cottage cheese, raspberries, and orange juice in food processor
until smooth. Refrigerate until ready to serve.
Serve with vanilla wafers.

Makes 2 cups or 8 servings.

1 serving (¼ cup) dip + 5 vanilla wafers = 1 starch/bread
+ 1 medium-fat protein + 2 fruit
Calories per serving = 290
Protein 8 g
Carbohydrates 35 g
Fat 7 g
Sodium 254 mg
Cholesterol 5 mg

Kahlua Fudge Sauce

6 ounce bag semisweet chocolate pieces
¼ cup water
½ teaspoon instant coffee granules
2 tablespoons Kahlua (coffee-flavored liqueur) optional

Combine chocolate pieces, water, and coffee granules in microwave-proof bowl.
Heat on high 2 minutes. Stir to dissolve granules and chips.
Stir in liqueur. Heat 1 minute longer.
Serve warm over fresh fruit cup or as dipping sauce for
sponge cake or sugar cookies.

Makes ¾ cup or 3 servings.

1 serving (¼ cup) = 1 fruit + 1 fat
Calories per serving = 101
Protein 1 g
Carbohydrates 18 g
Fat 7 g
Sodium 61 mg
Cholesterol 0

Granola Blueberry Crisp

2 cups fresh or frozen blueberries
¼ cup maple syrup
½ teaspoon ground cinnamon
¼ teaspoon ground nutmeg
2 1.5-ounce granola bars
½ cup vanilla low-fat yogurt

Combine blueberries, maple syrup, cinnamon, and nutmeg in bowl.
Toss to mix. Pour into individual custard cups or
8-inch-square baking pan. Crumble granola bars over fruit mixture.
Bake in preheated 350°F oven 20 to 25 minutes or until bubbly,
or microwave in glass baking dish on high 5 minutes until bubbly.
Serve with spoonful of yogurt on top.

Makes 4 servings.

1 serving = 2 fruit + 1 starch/bread + 1 fat
Calories per serving = 241
Protein 4 g
Carbohydrates 56 g
Fat 4 g
Sodium 94 mg
Cholesterol 26 mg

Chapter 6

Menus Featuring
Prepared Foods

Menus

Americans may be eating less total fat today than 10 years ago, but saturated fat and sodium are important to watch when selecting convenience meals. Our lifestyles have resulted in eating fewer fruits and vegetables, except salads and potatoes.

These menus are designed to provide healthy choices among available convenience items found in local supermarkets. Selections were made based on

- Fewer than 1,500 calories per day
- Sodium levels less than 4 grams (4,000 milligrams) per day
- Moderate intake of sugars from prepared foods
- Coffee, tea, diet soft drinks, or water as a beverage
- Total fat 25 to 35 percent of calories
- Total carbohydrates per meal and per day relatively consistent to assist those counting carbohydrates

Breakfast on the Run

- Choose a cereal, not a dessert. One cup of cereal with
  5 teaspoons of sugar = 10 Hershey Kisses! Make sure that your
  choice has less than 2 teaspoons sugar and no more than 100
  milligrams sodium per cup and is made from whole grains.
- Low-fat oatmeal cookies can substitute for oatmeal.
- Low-fat breakfast bars made from whole grains are easy
  to munch.
- Low-sugar, jam-filled pastries fit into pockets. (In years past,
  many were "candy bars," but they are lower in sugar and
  fat now.)
- Leftover turkey breast or chicken made into a sandwich can
  be easily consumed.

Day 1

		Calories	Total Fat (g)	Sodium (mg)	Carbo-hydrates (g)
Breakfast					
Cheerios, 1 cup		110	2	280	23
Low-fat (2%) milk, 1 cup		130	5	120	12
Orange juice, 1 cup		56	0	1	17
	Total	**296**	**7**	**401**	**52**
Lunch					
Burger King Whopper Jr., 1		420	24	530	29
No-calorie beverage (water, coffee, tea, diet soft drink)		0	0	0	0
	Total	**420**	**24**	**530**	**29**
Dinner					
Stouffer's Lean Cuisine lasagna		290	6	560	37
European salad greens: romaine & green leaf lettuce, 1½ cups		15	0	10	6
Good Seasons Italian fat-free dressing, 2 tablespoons		10	0	290	3
No-calorie beverage (water, coffee, tea, diet soft drink)		0	0	0	0
	Total	**315**	**6**	**860**	**45**
Snack					
Hostess Oat Bran Muffin, 1		160	8	224	9
Banana, 1 medium		105	1	1	27
	Total	**265**	**9**	**225**	**36**
DAILY TOTALS		**1,296**	**46**	**2,016**	**163**

Day 2

	Calories	Total Fat (g)	Sodium (mg)	Carbo-hydrates (g)
Breakfast				
McDonald's Egg McMuffin, 1	290	12	710	27
Orange juice, ½ cup	56	0	1	17
No-calorie beverage (water, coffee, tea, diet soft drink)	0	0	0	0
Total	346	12	711	44
Lunch				
Healthy Choice Mediterranean Bean with Pasta soup (canned), 2 cups	240	3	960	44
Dole Verona Salad: butter lettuce, radicchio, and frisee, 1½ cups	10	0	5	5
Seven Seas Viva Italian, 2 tablespoons	90	9	380	2
No-calorie beverage (water, coffee, tea, diet soft drink)	0	0	0	0
Total	340	12	1,345	51
Dinner				
Mrs. Paul's Grilled Salmon, 1	90	2	200	0
Birds Eye Roasted Potatoes & Broccoli, ⅔ cup	100	4	470	36
Breyers Natural Vanilla Ice Cream, ½ cup	150	9	53	15
No-calorie beverage (water, coffee, tea, diet soft drink)	0	0	0	0
Total	340	15	723	51
Snack				
Nabisco Chips Ahoy Cookies, 3	160	8	156	20
Low-fat (2%) milk, 1 cup	130	5	120	12
Total	290	13	276	32
DAILY TOTALS	1,316	52	3,055	178

Day 3

	Calories	Total Fat (g)	Sodium (mg)	Carbo-hydrates (g)
Breakfast				
Corn flakes, 1 cup	100	0	290	25
Low-fat (2%) milk, 1 cup	130	5	120	12
Nabisco Fat-Free Fig Newtons, 2	100	0	120	14
No-calorie beverage (water,				
coffee, tea, diet soft drink)	0	0	0	0
Total	330	5	530	51
Lunch				
Stouffer's Lean Cuisine				
Macaroni & Cheese, 1 package	290	7	630	42
Green Giant Broccoli, Cauliflower,				
Carrots & Cheese, ⅔ cup	80	3	570	11
No-calorie beverage (water,				
coffee, tea, diet soft drink)	0	0	0	0
Total	370	10	1,200	53
Dinner				
Birds Eye Shrimp Voila!				
Garlic Shrimp, 1 cup	230	9	590	27
Italian Bread, 1 slice	81	1	175	15
American salad blend:				
iceberg, romaine, carrots, 1½ cups	15	0	10	3
Hidden Valley Caesar Salad Dressing,				
2 tablespoons	110	11	290	1
No-calorie beverage (water,				
coffee, tea, diet soft drink)	0	0	0	0
Total	436	21	1,065	46
Snack				
Choice Food Bar	140	5	60	17
Apple, 1 medium	81	1	0	21
No-calorie beverage (water,				
coffee, tea, diet soft drink)	0	0	0	0
Total	221	6	60	38
DAILY TOTALS	1,357	47	2,855	176

Day 4

	Calories	Total Fat (g)	Sodium (mg)	Carbo- hydrates (g)
Breakfast				
Eggo Low-fat Blueberry				
Nutri-Grain Waffles, 2	160	2	420	30
Peanut butter, 1 tablespoon	95	8	80	3
Libby's Juicy Juice Punch, 4.23 oz.	80	0	0	19
Total	335	10	500	52
Lunch				
Tombstone Supreme Pizza,				
1 serving (130 grams)	330	17	670	35
No-calorie beverage (water,				
coffee, tea, diet soft drink)	0	0	0	0
Total	330	17	670	35
Dinner				
Green Giant Create a Meal Stir Fry:				
Cheesy Pasta & Vegetables,				
1¼ cups	420	21	1,350	48
European salad greens: romaine				
and green leaf lettuce, 1½ cups	15	0	10	6
Kraft Free Red Wine Vinegar,				
2 tablespoons	15	0	400	3
No-calorie beverage (water,				
coffee, tea, diet soft drink)	0	0	0	0
Total	450	21	1,760	57
Snack				
Hostess Cup Cake, 1, 2 oz.	180	6	176	17
Low-fat (2%) milk, 1 cup	130	5	120	12
Total	310	11	296	29
DAILY TOTALS	1,425	59	3,226	173

Day 5

	Calories	Total Fat (g)	Sodium (mg)	Carbo-hydrates (g)
Breakfast				
Aunt Jemima Cinnamon French Toast, 2	240	7	330	35
Bacon, 2 slices cooked	70	6	290	0
Mrs. Butterworth's Lite syrup, 1 fl. oz.	62	0	63	16
No-calorie beverage (water,				
coffee, tea, diet soft drink)	0	0	0	0
Total	**372**	**13**	**683**	**51**
Lunch				
Healthy Choice Turkey Divan	250	6	600	31
Green Giant Baby Brussels Sprouts				
and Butter, ½ cup	60	2	270	10
No-calorie beverage (water,				
coffee, tea, diet soft drink)	0	0	0	0
Total	**310**	**8**	**870**	**41**
Dinner				
Stouffer's Lean Cuisine Skillet				
Sensations: Herb Chicken	270	5	790	39
& Roasted Potatoes, 1½ cups				
Yoplait Lite Strawberry Yogurt, 6 fl. oz.	90	0	75	16
Banana, 1 medium	105	1	1	27
No-calorie beverage (water,				
coffee, tea, diet soft drink)	0	0	0	0
Total	**465**	**6**	**866**	**82**
Snack				
Entenmann's Light Cinnamon				
Bun, 2 oz.	160	3	250	17
No-calorie beverage (water,				
(coffee, tea, diet soft drink)	0	0	0	0
Total	**160**	**3**	**250**	**17**
DAILY TOTALS	**1,307**	**30**	**2,669**	**191**

Day 6

	Calories	Total Fat (g)	Sodium (mg)	Carbo-hydrates (g)
Breakfast				
Nutri-Grain Almond				
Raisin Cereal, ¾ cup	90	2	87	19
Yoplait Vanilla Yogurt, 6 fl. oz.	200	3	160	40
No-calorie beverage (water,				
coffee, tea, diet soft drink)	0	0	0	0
Total	**290**	**5**	**247**	**59**
Lunch				
Boston Market:				
¼ White Meat Chicken, low-fat				
w/o skin & wing	160	4	350	0
¾ cup Mediterranean Pasta Salad	170	10	490	16
¾ cup Fruit Salad, low-fat	70	1	10	17
No-calorie beverage (water,				
coffee, tea, diet soft drink)	0	0	0	0
Total	**400**	**15**	**850**	**33**
Dinner				
Weight Watchers Smart Ones:				
Ravioli Florentine	220	2	490	43
American salad blend:				
iceberg, romaine, carrots,				
1½ cups	15	0	10	3
Henri's Original French				
Salad Dressing, 2 tablespoons	120	11	200	6
No-calorie beverage (water,				
coffee, tea, diet soft drink)	0	0	0	0
Total	**355**	**13**	**700**	**52**
Snack				
Orange, 1 medium	60	0	1	15
Keebler Reduced-Fat				
Pecan Sandies, 2	140	6	180	6
Total	**200**	**6**	**181**	**21**
DAILY TOTALS	**1,245**	**39**	**1,978**	**165**

Day 7

		Calories	Total Fat (g)	Sodium (mg)	Carbo-hydrates (g)
Breakfast					
Pillsbury Cheese, Egg & Ham					
Toaster Sandwich, 1		180	12	350	15
Grapefruit juice, ½ cup		50	0	1	12
Low fat (2%) milk, 1 cup		130	5	120	12
	Total	360	17	471	39
Lunch					
Stouffer's Fish Filet with					
Macaroni & Cheese		430	21	930	12
Birds Eye Creamed Spinach, ½ cup		100	7	660	37
No-calorie beverage (water,					
coffee, tea, diet soft drink)		0	0	0	0
	Total	530	28	1,590	49
Dinner					
Progresso Minestrone					
99% Fat Free Soup, 1 cup		110	1	630	19
Healthy Choice Grilled					
Chicken Sonoma		230	4	530	30
No-calorie beverage (water,					
coffee, tea, diet soft drink)		0	0	0	0
	Total	340	5	1,160	49
Snack					
Pear, 1 medium raw		98	1	0	25
Entenmann's Light					
Blueberry Muffin, 1		120	0	251	15
No-calorie beverage (water,					
coffee, tea, diet soft drink)		0	0	0	0
	Total	218	1	251	40
DAILY TOTALS		1,448	51	3,472	177

Day 8

	Calories	Total Fat (g)	Sodium (mg)	Carbo-hydrates (g)
Breakfast				
General Mills Wheaties, 1 cup	110	1	220	24
Low-fat (2%) milk, 1 cup	130	5	120	12
Weight Watchers Smart Ones Muffin, 1	170	1	256	15
Total	**410**	**7**	**596**	**51**
Lunch				
Weight Watchers Smart Ones Spaghetti & Meat Sauce	280	5	670	43
American salad blend: iceberg, romaine, carrots, 1½ cups	15	0	10	3
Newman's Own Light Italian Salad Dressing, 2 tablespoons	45	4	370	3
No-calorie beverage (water, coffee, tea, diet soft drink)	0	0	0	0
Total	**340**	**9**	**1,050**	**49**
Dinner				
Gorton's Lemon Pepper Battered Fillets, 2	270	18	610	13
Lipton Noodles & Sauce Alfredo Broccoli, 1 cup	260	7	870	34
No-calorie beverage (water, coffee, tea, diet soft drink)	0	0	0	0
Total	**530**	**25**	**1,480**	**47**
Snack				
Apple, 1 medium	81	1	0	21
Total	**81**	**1**	**0**	**21**
DAILY TOTALS	**1,361**	**42**	**3,126**	**168**

Day 9

		Calories	Total Fat (g)	Sodium (mg)	Carbo-hydrates (g)
Breakfast					
Red Barron Breakfast Pizza:					
Ham Scramble, 1		360	17	780	35
No-calorie beverage (water,					
coffee, tea, diet soft drink)		0	0	0	0
	Total	360	17	780	35
Lunch					
Healthy Choice Roasted Chicken		230	5	480	25
Philadelphia Classic Cheesecake					
Snack Bar, 1		200	13	371	17
No-calorie beverage (water,					
coffee, tea, diet soft drink)		0	0	0	0
	Total	430	18	851	42
Dinner					
Chef's Choice Shrimp Linguini, 1 cup		180	1	720	28
French bread, 1 slice		81	0	163	15
No-calorie beverage (water,					
coffee, tea, diet soft drink)		0	0	0	0
	Total	261	1	883	43
Snack					
Banana milk shake:					
Banana, 1 medium		110	0	0	29
Low-fat (2%) milk, 1 cup		130	5	120	12
4–6 ice cubes		0	0	0	0
	Total	240	5	120	41
DAILY TOTALS		1,291	41	2,634	161

Day 10

	Calories	Total Fat (g)	Sodium (mg)	Carbo-hydrates (g)
Breakfast				
Swanson Scrambled Eggs & Sausage with Hash Browns, 1	360	26	800	20
No-calorie beverage (water, coffee, tea, diet soft drink)	0	0	0	0
Total	360	26	800	20
Lunch				
Ocean Beauty Tuna Burger, 1	90	1	340	6
French roll, 1	105	2	231	19
Tartar sauce, nonfat, 2 tablespoons	25	0	210	5
Light 'n Lively Yogurt, 4.4 fl. oz.	140	1	63	27
Strawberries, ½ cup	25	0	1	7
No-calorie beverage (water, coffee, tea, diet soft drink)	0	0	0	0
Total	385	4	845	64
Dinner				
Campbell's Healthy Request Soup: Hearty Chicken, 2 cups	200	4	720	32
Healthy Choice American Single Cheese, 2 slices	80	2	400	0
Saltine crackers, 5	65	2	195	11
No-calorie beverage (water, coffee, tea, diet soft drink)	0	0	0	0
Total	345	8	1,315	43
Snack				
Grapes, 1 cup	114	1	3	28
Nabisco Lorna Doone, 4	140	7	130	29
Total	254	8	133	57
DAILY TOTALS	1,344	46	3,093	184

Day 11

		Calories	Total Fat (g)	Sodium (mg)	Carbo- hydrates (g)
Breakfast					
Shredded wheat, 1 oz.		102	1	1	23
Low-fat (2%) milk, 1 cup		130	5	120	12
Banana, 1 medium		105	1	1	27
	Total	337	7	122	62
Lunch					
Subway Turkey Breast & Ham on white, 6 inches		280	5	1,350	39
Pear, 1 medium raw		98	1	0	25
No-calorie beverage (water, coffee, tea, diet soft drink)		0	0	0	0
	Total	378	6	1,350	64
Dinner					
Stouffer's Lean Cuisine Oven Roasted Beef		240	8	590	27
Cabbage & carrot salad, 1 cup		13	0	8	3
Kraft Cole Slaw Dressing, 2 tablespoons		130	11	410	7
No-calorie beverage (water, coffee, tea, diet soft drink)		0	0	0	0
	Total	383	19	1,008	37
Snack					
Pretzels, 1 oz.		108	1	486	23
No-calorie beverage (water, coffee, tea, diet soft drink)		0	0	0	0
	Total	108	1	486	23
DAILY TOTALS		1,206	33	2,966	186

Day 12

		Calories	Total Fat (g)	Sodium (mg)	Carbo-hydrates (g)
Breakfast					
English muffin, 1		134	1	264	26
Colby cheese, reduced fat, 2 oz.		160	12	440	0
Orange juice, ½ cup		56	0	1	17
	Total	**350**	**13**	**705**	**43**
Lunch					
Taco Bell Taco Salad w/salsa w/o shell		420	22	1,520	32
No-calorie beverage (water, coffee, tea, diet soft drink)		0	0	0	0
	Total	**420**	**22**	**1,520**	**32**
Dinner					
Birds Eye Chicken Voila!: Romano Herb Chicken w/Roasted Potatoes, 1½ cups		330	11	1,065	56
No-calorie beverage (water, (coffee, tea, diet soft drink)		0	0	0	0
	Total	**330**	**11**	**1,065**	**56**
Snack					
Milky Way, 1, 2.1 oz.		270	10	146	35
	Total	**270**	**10**	**146**	**35**
DAILY TOTALS		**1,370**	**56**	**3,436**	**166**

Day 13

	Calories	Total Fat (g)	Sodium (mg)	Carbo-hydrates (g)
Breakfast				
Hungry Jack Buttermilk Pancakes, 3	270	4	630	50
Mrs. Butterworth's Lite Syrup, 1 fl. oz.	62	0	63	16
No-calorie beverage (water,				
coffee, tea, diet soft drink)	0	0	0	0
Total	332	4	693	66
Lunch				
Stouffer's French Bread Pizza:				
Pepperoni (159 grams)	390	16	840	48
No-calorie beverage (water,				
coffee, tea, diet soft drink)	0	0	0	0
Total	390	16	840	48
Dinner				
Kraft Shake 'n Bake Glaze Tangy				
Honey (coating for 1 pork chop)	45	1	300	18
Pork chop, 3.5 oz.	232	11	86	0
Betty Crocker Creamy Herb				
Risotto Rice, ½ cup	185	4	380	20
Green beans, ½ cup	22	0	2	5
No-calorie beverage (water,				
coffee, tea, diet soft drink)	0	0	0	0
Total	484	16	768	43
Snack				
Strawberry banana yogurt shake:				
Yoplait Lite Strawberry Yogurt,				
6 fl. oz.	90	1	1	14
Banana, ½ medium	55	0	0	15
4–6 ice cubes	0	0	0	0
Total	145	1	1	29
DAILY TOTALS	1,351	37	2,302	186

Day 14

	Calories	Total Fat (g)	Sodium (mg)	Carbo-hydrates (g)
Breakfast				
SnackWell's Oatmeal Raisin Cookies, 4	240	6	120	20
Low-fat (2%) milk, 1 cup	130	5	120	12
Total	370	11	240	32
Lunch				
Wendy's Grilled Chicken Sandwich, 1	310	8	790	35
Potato chips, 1 oz.	152	10	168	15
No-calorie beverage (water, coffee, tea, diet soft drink)	0	0	0	0
Total	462	18	958	50
Dinner				
Van de Kamp's Crispy Battered Ocean Perch Fillets, 2	240	13	510	19
Betty Crocker Garlic Alfredo Fettucine Pasta, 1 cup	220	3	700	35
Chopped spinach, ½ cup	21	0	63	3
No-calorie beverage (water, coffee, tea, diet soft drink)	0	0	0	0
Total	481	16	1,273	57
Snack				
Häagen-Dazs Low-Fat Chocolate Ice Cream, ½ cup	170	3	57	15
Total	170	3	57	15
DAILY TOTALS	1,483	48	2,528	154

Chapter 7
Prepared–Food Comparisons

---

*F*rozen dinners have been viewed as the worst form of prepared foods available today. American lifestyles and nutritional demands, however, have led some manufacturers to provide convenience with fewer "nasty" ingredients (fat and sugar). This menu book is written to help you make the healthiest choices from currently available prepared foods. One way of getting healthier convenience foods is to compare brands and buy those with less fat, sugar, and sodium.

Soups and sauces are another big convenience item on the menu. Some manufacturers offer good variety with low fat and low sodium. Fresh or frozen vegetables can be added to make a more nutritious meal choice.

Prepared salad dressings are hardly a new convenience item in the daily menu. Many low-fat versions are available in shelf-stable and refrigerated varieties. Always remember to store them in the refrigerator after opening and use within a 2- to 3-month period.

Let your fingers do the walking through these prepared-foods comparisons. Enjoy the convenience of selecting the best choice *before* you arrive at the supermarket. Why stand in front of the frozen-food case trying to decide which pizza or skillet meal has less sodium and fat? You can do it when sitting in your living room.

These listings are not inclusive of every brand name in the super-market. They are a representation of the variety of products currently available. Nutrient values have been rounded to whole numbers for easier comparison.

Cereals

When it comes to planning breakfast, cereal is usually the fast and easy choice. Whole grain cereals without the "breakfast candy" amount of sugar are the recommended nutritional choice.

Brand	Name	Amount	Calories	Sugar (g)
General Mills	Basic 4	1 cup	200	14
	Cheerios	1 cup	110	1
	Cocoa Puffs	1 cup	120	14
	Corn Chex	1 cup	110	3
	Crispy Wheaties 'N Raisins	1 cup	190	20
	Fiber One	½ cup	60	0
	Frosted Cheerios	1 cup	120	13
	Honey Frosted Wheaties	¾ cup	110	12
	Honey Nut Cheerios	1 cup	120	11
	Kix	1⅓ cups	120	3
	Lucky Charms	1 cup	120	13
	Multi-Bran Chex	1 cup	200	12
	MultiGrain Cheerios Plus	1 cup	110	6
	Oatmeal Crisp, Almond	1 cup	220	15
	Oatmeal Crisp, Apple Cinnamon	1 cup	210	19
	Raisin Nut Bran	¾ cup	200	16
	Rice Chex	1¼ cups	120	2
	Toasted Oatmeal Squares	1 cup	220	9
	Total Corn Flakes	1⅓ cups	110	3
	Total Raisin Bran	1 cup	180	19
	Trix	1 cup	120	13
	Wheat Chex	1 cup	180	1
	Wheaties	1 cup	110	4
	Whole Grain Total	¾ cup	110	5

Brand	Name	Amount	Calories	Sugar (g)
Healthy Choice	Almond Crunch with Raisins	1 cup	210	15
	Apple & Almond Crunch Mueslix	⅔ cup	200	12
	Golden Multi Grain Flakes	¾ cup	110	6
	Low-Fat Granola	⅓ cup	190	14
	Low-Fat Granola with Raisins	⅔ cup	220	16
	Toasted Brown Sugar Squares	1 cup	190	9
Kellogg's	All-Bran	⅔ cup	80	6
	All-Bran Bran Buds	½ cup	80	8
	Apple Jacks	1 cup	120	16
	Bite Size Frosted Mini Wheats	24 biscuits	200	12
	Cocoa Krispies	¾ cup	120	14
	Corn Flakes	1 cup	100	2
	Corn Pops	1 cup	120	14
	Cracklin' Oat Bran	¾ cup	190	15
	Ensemble	1 cup	120	10
	Frosted Flakes	¾ cup	120	13
	Fruit Loops	1 cup	120	15
	Honey Crunch Corn Flakes	¾ cup	120	10
	Nutri-Grain Almond Raisin	1¼ cups	180	7
	Nutri-Grain Golden Wheat	¾ cup	100	0
	Product 19	1 cup	100	4
	Raisin Bran	1 cup	200	18
	Rice Krispies	1¼ cups	120	3
	Rice Krispies Treats Cereal	¾ cup	120	9
	Smart Start	1 cup	180	15
	Special K	1 cup	110	4
Post	100% Bran	⅓ cup	80	7
	Alpha-Bits	1 cup	130	12
	Bran Flakes	¾ cup	100	6
	Cocoa Puffs	¾ cup	120	13
	Fruit & Fibre	1 cup	210	16
	Fruity Pebbles	¾ cup	110	12
	Grape-Nuts	½ cup	200	7
	Grape-Nuts Flakes	¾ cup	100	5
	Honeycomb	1⅓ cups	110	11
	Oreo O's	¾ cup	110	11
	Raisin Bran	1 cup	190	20
	Shredded Wheat	2 biscuits	160	0

Continued overleaf

Brand	Name	Amount	Calories	Sugar (g)
Post, *cont.*	Shredded Wheat 'N Bran	1¼ cups	200	0
	Spoon-Size Shredded Wheat	1 cup	170	0
	Toasties	1 cup	100	2
Quaker	100% Natural Granola	½ cup	220	15
	100% Natural Low-Fat Granola	⅔ cup	210	18
	Cap'N Crunch	¾ cup	110	11
	Crunchy Corn Bran	¾ cup	90	6
	Life	¾ cup	120	8
	Oat Bran	1¼ cups	210	9
	Shredded Wheat	3 biscuits	220	1
	Sun Country Granola	½ cup	270	15
	Toasted Almond Squares	1 cup	220	9

Frozen Breakfast Items

Whether one eats breakfast at the crack of dawn or midmorning, everyone needs to replenish their body's store of glucose after an 8- to 10-hour fast. Research has shown how breakfast enhances mental and physical performances at all ages. If you think about skipping breakfast because there isn't enough time, keep some quick and easy breakfast foods on hand. Cereal and milk, toaster waffles with turkey sausage, or leftovers from dinner all qualify as "breakfast food."

Ready-to-eat breakfast meals offer convenience with a substantial amount of calories, fat, and sodium. Use of these products can be an occasional treat when the rest of the day's menu features low-fat, low-sodium selections.

Many of the convenience breakfast items—pancakes, waffles, French toast—have significant levels of carbohydrates *without* syrup. To keep the carbohydrates in the breakfast meal and under control, use low-calorie/sugar-free syrup, applesauce, or a sugar-free fruit spread. Pass on adding any extra butter or margarine.

Brand	Amount	Calories	Fat (g)	Sodium (mg)	Carbohy-drates (g)
Frozen Breakfast Meals					
Croissant Pockets:					
Egg, Sausage & Cheese	1	340	15	740	40
Pillsbury Toaster Scrambles:					
Cheese & Egg	1	170	11	330	15
Cheese, Egg & Bacon	1	180	12	360	15
Cheese, Egg & Ham	1	180	12	350	15
Cheese, Egg & Sausage	1	180	12	350	15
Red Barron Breakfast Pizza:					
Bacon Scramble	1	440	25	980	35
Ham Scramble	1	360	17	780	35
Western Scramble	1	400	22	820	35
Swanson Bacon Burrito	1	250	10	540	30
Swanson Egg, Cheese &					
Bacon on Biscuit	1	350	20	890	30
Swanson Scrambled Eggs &					
Sausage w/Hash Browns	1	360	26	800	20
French Toast, Pancakes, Waffles					
Aunt Jemima:					
Buttermilk Waffles	2	200	6	550	30
Cinnamon French Toast	2	240	7	330	35
Cinnamon French					
Toast Sticks	4	350	13	520	50
Lowfat Pancakes	3	150	1	530	30
Lowfat Waffles	2	160	1	540	30
Mini Pancakes	13	240	4	640	45
Eggo:					
Blueberry Waffles	2	200	7	420	30
Buttermilk Pancakes	3	270	8	610	45
Buttermilk Waffles	2	190	7	420	30
Low-Fat Blueberry					
Nutri-Grain Waffles	2	150	2	420	30
Low-Fat Homestyle Waffles	2	160	2	300	30
Nutri-Grain Waffles	2	170	5	420	30
Hungry Jack:					
Blueberry Pancakes	3	240	4	550	50
Blueberry Waffles	2	210	7	540	30
Buttermilk Pancakes	3	270	4	630	50
Buttermilk Waffles	2	190	6	530	30

Fruit Juice and Drinks

Fruit beverages labeled "juice" must be 100% juice. A fruit juice "beverage," "punch," "drink," or "cocktail" can contain little juice and lots of water plus sugar. The amount of actual fruit juice in a drink product can be anywhere from 1 to 40 percent.

This fruit juice and drinks listing provides calories and total carbohydrates in a serving. Because the American Diabetes Association guidelines recommend monitoring total carbohydrates instead of the type of sugar in the diet, simple sugars are not listed separately.

Research has shown that what affects blood glucose is the total amount of sugar *or total carbohydrates* in a serving of juice, *not the type of sugar* in the juice. The more sugar added to a fruit drink, the higher the calories and carbohydrates.

Brand	Flavor	Amount	Calories	Carbohy- drates (g)
Capri Sun	All-Natural Juice Pouches:			
	Grape, Orange	6.75 oz.	100	25
	Wild Cherry	6.75 oz.	100	30
Dole	Pineapple	6 oz.	80	22
	Pine-Orange Banana	8 oz.	120	29
Hawaiian Punch	Blue Cooler	6.75 oz.	100	26
Hi C	Boppin' Berry Orange	6.75 oz.	100	27
	Fruit Juicy Red	8 oz.	120	30
	Orange Drink	8 oz.	120	32
Kool-Aid	Bursts	6.75 oz.	100	24
Libby's	Juicy Juice:			
	Apple	8 oz.	120	29
	Punch	4.23 oz.	80	19
	Tropical	8.45 oz.	140	34
Minute Maid	Apple	6.75 oz.	90	23
	Five Alive	8 oz.	120	30
	Grape	6.75 oz.	100	26
	Lemonade	8 oz.	110	31

Brand	Flavor	Amount	Calories	Carbohy-drates (g)
	Orange	8 oz.	110	27
	Tropical Punch	6.75 oz.	100	26
Mott's	Apple	8 oz.	120	29
	Fruit Punch	8 oz.	120	30
	Grape	8 oz.	120	31
Ocean Spray	100% Juice Pink Grapefruit	8 oz.	110	28
	Cranapple	8 oz.	160	41
	Cranapple Reduced Calorie	8 oz.	50	13
	Cranberry Juice Cocktail	8 oz.	140	34
	Cranberry Juice Cocktail Reduced Calorie	8 oz.	50	13
	Crangrape	8 oz.	170	41
R W Knudsen	Organic Pear	8 oz.	120	30
Sunsweet	Prune	8 oz.	170	42
Tropicana	Golden Grapefruit	8 oz.	90	22
	Orange	8 oz.	110	26
Welch's	100% Grape	8 oz.	170	42

Salads

Fresh packaged salad greens are quickly replacing cabbage shredders and cutting boards. These greens are prewashed, so they only need a bowl for serving up a variety of salad choices for lunch and dinner. Shredded cabbage and carrot mixtures are making heads of cabbage obsolete in the produce section of the supermarket.

Pasta salad mixes can make a quick meal accompaniment. Leftovers with some chicken or tuna can make for a tasty lunch the next day.

As in any salad choice, the dressing makes a lot of difference. Prepared salad dressings are convenient, and many reduced-calorie or fat-free varieties help keep calories and fat under control.

Brand	Serving Size	Calories	Fat (g)	Sodium (mg)
Salad Blends				
Fresh Express:				
American: iceberg, romaine, carrots	1½ cups	15	0	10
Cabbage and carrots	2 cups	25	0	15
European: romaine, & green leaf	1½ cups	15	0	10
Dole Verona:				
Butter lettuce, radicchio, & frisee	1½ cups	10	0	5
Pasta Salad Mixes				
Betty Crocker Suddenly Salad:				
Classic	¾ cup	250	8	910
Ranch & bacon	¾ cup	330	20	480
Kraft Pasta Salad:				
Creamy Caesar	¾ cup	340	21	630
97% Fat-Free Italian	¾ cup	190	2	740

Salad Dressings

Gone are the days when salad dressing was known as mayonnaise or oil and vinegar. The hundreds of commercially prepared salad dressings range from traditional French and Italian to thousand island, blue cheese, and raspberry vinaigrette.

The main ingredient (except fat-free varieties) of salad dressing is oil. This concentrated source of calories requires prudence when deciding how much dressing to pour onto your salad greens. Two tablespoons is a usual portion, but many people use considerably more. Drowning vegetables in lots of fat is not a healthy choice.

Generally speaking, oil and vinegar-type dressings (Italian, raspberry vinaigrette) have less fat per serving than creamy dressings (ranch, blue cheese, thousand island). In addition, thinner-type dressings coat the lettuce leaves and then sink to the bottom of the bowl or plate. Creamy dressings adhere to lettuce leaves, and you end up reaching for more dressing to finish eating the greens.

Reduced-calorie or fat-free varieties feature low fat content, but they are not calorie free. Many of these dressings have sugar, food starches, and extra sodium to make up for the flavor lost from omitting higher-calorie ingredients.

Another convenient use of prepared salad dressings is to use them as a basting sauce or marinade for meat, poultry, or fish. They add flavor to steamed vegetables and make a quick snack dip.

Brand	Variety	Serving Size	Calories	Fat (g)	Sodium (mg)	Carbohy-drates (g)
Good Seasons	Gourmet Caesar	2 tbsp.	150	16	300	3
	Italian	2 tbsp.	190	15	320	1
	Italian Fat-Free	2 tbsp.	10	0	290	3

Continued overleaf

Brand	Variety	Serving Size	Calories	Fat (g)	Sodium (mg)	Carbohy-drates (g)
Hellman's	Creamy Ranch	2 tbsp.	140	15	320	1
	Creamy 1,000 Island	2 tbsp.	130	13	270	4
	Fat-Free French	2 tbsp.	45	0	260	12
	Fat-Free Ranch	2 tbsp.	45	0	380	11
Henri's	Balsamic Vinaigrette					
	Fat-Free	2 tbsp.	15	0	300	4
	Cream Caesar Fat-Free	2 tbsp.	45	0	300	11
	French Fat-Free	2 tbsp.	45	0	240	11
	Original French	2 tbsp.	120	11	200	6
Hidden Valley	Caesar	2 tbsp.	110	11	290	1
	Fat-Free Ranch					
	w/Bacon	2 tbsp.	50	0	340	11
	Light Ranch	2 tbsp.	80	7	270	3
	Original Ranch	2 tbsp.	140	14	260	1
Kraft	Catalina	2 tbsp.	130	11	410	8
	Catalina (Light)	2 tbsp.	70	5	400	9
	Coleslaw	2 tbsp.	130	11	410	7
	Cucumber Ranch	2 tbsp.	140	15	220	2
	Free Blue Cheese	2 tbsp.	45	0	340	11
	Free Ranch	2 tbsp.	50	0	350	11
	Free Red Wine Vinegar	2 tbsp.	15	0	400	3
	Thousand Island	2 tbsp.	110	10	310	5
	Thousand Island (Light)	2 tbsp.	70	4	300	7
Newman's	Light Italian	2 tbsp.	45	4	370	3
Own	Olive Oil & Vinegar	2 tbsp.	150	16	150	1
	Ranch	2 tbsp.	140	15	250	2
Seven Seas	Green Goddess	2 tbsp.	130	13	260	1
	Viva Italian	2 tbsp.	90	9	380	2
Wish-Bone	Chunky Blue Cheese	2 tbsp.	170	17	280	2
	Fat-Free Chunky Blue					
	Cheese	2 tbsp.	35	0	290	7
	Fat-Free French	2 tbsp.	30	0	230	7
	Italian	2 tbsp.	80	8	490	3
	Lite Italian	2 tbsp.	15	1	500	2
	Russian	2 tbsp.	110	6	350	15

Complete Prepared Meals

Whether you refer to them as frozen dinners or as complete all-in-one meals, it makes little difference. The food industry refers to them as home meal replacements, because these convenience products are rapidly changing how Americans eat.

It doesn't get much easier than standing in front of the frozen-food case or refrigerated take-out area of the supermarket. The only planning necessary is to determine which cuisine appeals to the appetite and pocketbook. Stopping at the supermarket for a prepared meal or briefcase salad on the way to work in the morning solves the lunch dilemma. Others pick up a can of soup for a fast meal that requires no refrigeration, but canned soups are very high in sodium compared with the fresh and frozen meal choices. It would be quite difficult to stay under the 1,000 milligrams sodium per meal and select most of the canned soups listed.

Brand	Calories	Fat (g)	Sodium (mg)	Carbohy-drates (g)
Fresh Food				
Harry's Farmers Market, Roswell, GA:				
Biryani Rice	210	6	620	37
Caesar Salad - Briefcase Salad	210	18	430	7
Cheese Lasagna	340	15	710	29
Grilled Beef Sirloin with Vegetables	300	8	290	26
Grilled Chicken with Vegetables	260	5	290	26
Grilled Chicken Breast with Salsa Fresca and Broccoli Rice	290	5	890	24
Macaroni and Cheese	430	26	900	30
Manicotti	310	13	660	32
Roast Turkey and Dressing w/ Gravy and Carrots	710	27	2180	57
Roasted Salmon with Vegetables	280	8	280	27

Continued overleaf

Brand	Calories	Fat (g)	Sodium (mg)	Carbohy-drates (g)
Frozen Choices				
Amy's Kitchen (Vegetarian, Organic):				
Broccoli Pot Pie w/Cheddar Cheese Sauce	430	22	630	46
Country Vegetable Pie	370	16	580	47
Vegetable Lasagna	300	10	680	39
Veggie Loaf, Mashed Potatoes, & Vegetables	260	5	690	47
Budget Gourmet:				
Beef Stroganoff	240	6	690	32
Chicken & Egg Noodles	370	21	760	31
Roast Beef Supreme	270	10	690	34
Three Cheese Lasagna	320	13	700	35
Healthy Choice:				
Beef Pot Roast	330	9	600	41
Breaded Chicken Breast Strips w/ Macaroni & Cheese	270	5	600	34
Charbroiled Beef Patty	310	9	550	40
Cheesy Rice & Chicken	250	3	600	45
Chicken Broccoli Alfredo	300	7	530	34
Chicken Enchilada	310	7	600	46
Chicken Fettuccini Alfredo	280	7	600	30
Chicken Parmigiana	320	9	600	40
Chicken Teriyaki w/Rice	270	4	570	41
Country Breaded Chicken	380	8	450	57
Fiesta Chicken	220	2	550	34
Grilled Chicken Breast & Pasta	240	6	600	26
Grilled Chicken Sonoma	230	4	530	30
Hearty Handfuls Turkey & Vegetables	310	5	560	51
Mesquite Chicken BBQ	290	5	550	45
Oven Roasted Chicken	280	7	600	32
Roasted Chicken	230	5	480	25
Sesame Chicken	250	4	600	38
Southwestern Style Rice & Beans	230	4	600	34
Turkey Divan	250	6	600	31
Living Well:				
Herb Roasted Chicken	220	5	350	31

Brand	Calories	Fat (g)	Sodium (mg)	Carbohy-drates (g)
Marie Callender:				
Turkey Pot Pie	690	46	1,100	56
Michelina's Signature:				
Chicken Marsala	280	1	980	22
Meatloaf	340	23	1,230	20
Roasted Sirloin Supreme	280	10	1,230	34
Stouffer's Lean Cuisine:				
Baked Chicken Florentine	220	5	640	32
Baked Fish w/Cheddar Shells	290	6	650	40
Chicken Carbonara	280	7	560	36
Chicken Piccata	270	6	530	41
Glazed Chicken	330	8	840	34
Lasagna	290	6	560	37
Lasagna w/Seasoned Meat Sauce	300	8	570	35
Meatloaf	260	7	600	28
Oven Roasted Beef	240	8	590	27
Roasted Potatoes, Broccoli & Cheese Sauce	260	6	590	39
Sante Fe Style Rice & Beans	300	5	650	54
Spaghetti w/Meat Balls & Sauce	270	6	590	37
Swedish Meatballs w/Pasta	290	7	690	35
Stouffer's:				
Cheddar Cheese & Chicken Bake	450	21	1,230	41
Chicken Parmigiana	460	16	1,060	54
Chunky Beef & Tomatoes	280	9	1,480	33
Fish Filet w/ Macaroni & Cheese	430	21	930	37
Five Cheese Lasagna	360	13	960	40
Lasagna w/Meat & Sauce	370	14	1,050	39
Macaroni & Beef w/Tomatoes	380	15	1,210	37
Thai Chef:				
Lemongrass & Basil Chicken	390	10	105	55
Peanut Satay Chicken	400	14	740	50

Continued overleaf

Brand	Calories	Fat (g)	Sodium (mg)	Carbohy-drates (g)
Weight Watchers Smart Ones:				
Grilled Salisbury Steak & Gravy w/				
Macaroni & Cheese	290	8	770	29
Lasagna Bolognese	240	3	560	43
Slow Roasted Turkey Breast	220	7	660	20

Canned Products

Brand	Calories	Fat (g)	Sodium (mg)	Carbohy-drates (g)
Campbell's Chunky Soups:				
Beef w/Country Vegetables (1 can)	190	5	1,130	22
Hearty Chicken w/				
Vegetables (2 cups)	180	4	1,600	24
Savory Chicken w/				
White & Wild Rice (2 cups)	280	6	1,680	36
Sirloin Burger w/				
Country Vegetables (1 can)	250	11	1,250	22
Steak 'N Potato (2 cups)	300	8	1,780	38
Campbell's Healthy Request Soups:				
Hearty Chicken Rice (2 cups)	200	4	720	32
Split Pea w/Ham (2 cups)	340	3	720	58
Classico It's Pasta Anytime:				
Penne w/Tomato Italian				
Sausage-Flavored Sauce	540	8	850	100
Spaghetti Style Pasta w/				
Tomato Beef-Flavored Sauce	540	8	890	101
Healthy Choice Soups:				
Chicken Alfredo Style (2 cups)	220	3	960	40
Hearty Chicken (2 cups)	260	4	960	42
Mediterranean Bean w/Pasta (2 cups)	240	3	960	44
Progresso Soups:				
Beefy Barley 99% Fat-Free (2 cups)	260	4	1,420	40
Minestrone 99% Fat-Free (2 cups)	220	2	1,260	38
Turkey Noodle (2 cups)	180	3	2,120	22

Bowl Products

Brand	Calories	Fat (g)	Sodium (mg)	Carbohy-drates (g)
Betty Crocker Bowl Appetit:				
Tomato Parmesan Penne	350	8	890	57
Healthy Choice Bowls:				
Turkey Divan	270	7	600	30

Brand	Calories	Fat (g)	Sodium (mg)	Carbohy- drates (g)
Uncle Ben's Noodle Bowl:				
Spicy Thai Style Chicken	400	8	980	60
Weight Watchers:				
Beef & Vegetable Rice Bowl	260	5	790	40
Vegetarian Choices				
Tasty Bite:				
Bengal Lentils	190	5	150	30
Bombay Potatoes	190	8	720	22
Jaipur Vegetables	220	15	680	13
Kashmir Spinach	170	10	960	8
Punjab Eggplant	130	8	780	9

Main-Dish Kits

The *almost* complete meal offers another option for a quick dinner when schedules have run late or you have barely enough energy to fix a grilled cheese sandwich. These meal kits come usually at a high cost in dollars and lots of sodium. Adding a salad or extra vegetable can make a satisfying meal—for most people—with adequate leftovers for a quick lunch the next day. These meal kits require the addition of chicken, meat, or fish. Read the label closely to notice how complete it is.

Trying to keep the sodium level per meal to 500 to 1,000 milligrams will be difficult with some of these main-dish kits, so make your choices wisely.

Brand	Serving Size	Calories	Fat (g)	Sodium (mg)
Skillet & Stir-Fry Meal Kits (add chicken, meat, or other protein source)				
Birds Eye Easy Recipe Creations:				
Basil Herb Primavera	1½ cups	440	15	890
Oriental Lo Mein	1½ cups	360	5	1,200
Roasted Garlic Parmesan	1½ cups	400	13	820
Sesame Ginger Teriyaki	1½ cups	270	4	1,230
Sweet & Sour	1½ cups	330	3	360
Tortellini Parmigiana	1½ cups	410	16	960
Cascadian Farm Quickstart:				
South Indian Curry	2½ cups	260	8	620
Teriyaki Veggies & Rice	2¼ cups	290	10	650
Thai Veggies & Rice	2¼ cups	270	7	470
Green Giant Create a Meal Stir Fry:				
Beef & Broccoli	1⅓ cups	250	8	1,150
Beefy Noodle	1¼ cups	350	14	1,130
Cheesy Pasta & Vegetables	1¼ cups	420	21	1,350
Chicken Alfredo	1¼ cups	360	8	1,100
Garlic & Ginger	1½ cups	230	2	1,130
Garlic Herb Chicken	1¼ cups	340	10	870
Homestyle Stew	1 cup	340	16	1,370
Lo Mein	1¼ cups	280	2	920
Mushroom Wine Chicken	1¼ cups	350	8	1,110
Skillet Lasagna	1¼ cups	340	13	830
Sweet and Sour	1¼ cups	300	2	620
Szechuan	1¼ cups	270	9	1,390
Teriyaki	1¼ cups	190	1	920

Brand	Serving Size	Calories	Fat (g)	Sodium (mg)
Oven Roasted Kits (add chicken)				
Green Giant Create a Meal Oven Roasted:				
Barbecue Chicken	1½ cups	350	9	1,340
Chicken and Stuffing	1½ cups	370	11	1,540
Garlic Herb Chicken	1¾ cups	350	9	760
Lemon Pepper Chicken	1⅔ cups	310	8	1,400
Parmesan Herb Chicken	1¾ cups	340	11	1,050

Frozen Seafood Items

Seafood offers omega-3 fatty acids, which research has indicated can reduce the risk of sudden death heart attacks. Eating at least two fish meals a week is recommended as good protection for the heart. Fatty fish like salmon, sardines, herring, and trout have more omega-3 fatty acids, but any fish (flounder, haddock, sole, etc.) may also be eaten as part of a healthy heart diet.

The fried, breaded, and stuffed selections listed below have significantly higher levels of total fat than unbreaded fillets. Sodium levels can be twice as high in breaded selections. Stocking the freezer with some of these fish choices can provide a quick and healthy meal.

Brand	Amount	Calories	Fat (g)	Sodium (mg)
Unbreaded fillets				
Galletti Brothers:				
Alaskan Cod Fillets	4 oz.	90	0	70
Alaskan Halibut Steaks	4 oz.	130	3	60
Orange Roughy Fillets	4 oz.	140	8	70
Pacific Red Snapper Fillets	4 oz.	110	2	105

Continued overleaf

Brand	Amount	Calories	Fat (g)	Sodium (mg)
Gorton's:				
Gorton's Grilled Salmon	3 oz.	110	5	390
Grilled Fillets	1	110	5	270
Mrs. Paul's:				
Grilled Fillets	1	130	6	260
Grilled Salmon	1	90	2	200
Sea Best:				
Alaska Pollock	4 oz.	110	1	140
Arrowtooth Flounder	4 oz.	125	2	110
Van de Kamp's:				
Grilled Fillets	1	120	6	200

Breaded/Battered/Stuffed Fillets

Brand	Amount	Calories	Fat (g)	Sodium (mg)
Gorton's:				
Baked Fillets	1	140	6	350
Crispy Battered Fish Fillets	2	250	15	540
Crunchy Breaded Fish Fillets	2	250	14	620
Crunchy Golden Fish Fillets	2	260	16	350
Crunchy Stuff Fillets	1	270	13	560
Lemon Pepper Battered Fillets	2	270	18	610
Mrs. Paul's:				
Healthy Selects Baked Fish Fillets	1	130	2	330
Select Cuts Cod Fillets	1	260	14	350
Select Cuts Crispy Battered Fish Fillets	1	200	10	510
Select Cuts Crispy Fish Fillets	2	280	18	430
Select Cuts Haddock Fillets	1	240	12	330
Van de Kamp's:				
Crisp and Healthy Fish Fillets	2	170	3	430
Crispy Battered Fish Fillets	1	170	10	390
Crispy Battered Haddock Fillets	2	240	12	530
Crispy Battered Halibut Fillets	3	220	10	530
Crispy Battered Ocean Perch Fillets	2	240	13	510
Crispy Breaded Fish Portions	3	360	24	480
Crispy Fish Fillets	2	300	20	440
Crispy Flounder Fillets	1	230	11	390
Crispy Haddock Fillets	1	230	11	410

Brand	Amount	Calories	Fat (g)	Sodium (mg)
Burgers				
Aqua Cuisine:				
Salmon Burger	1	90	0	210
Ocean Beauty:				
Salmon Burger	1	80	1	310
Tuna Burger	1	90	1	340
Trader Joe's:				
Premium Salmon Patties	1	80	1	320
Shellfish (crab, scallops, shrimp)				
Gorton's:				
Popcorn Shrimp	24	290	14	970
Popcorn Shrimp, Garlic & Herb	24	270	13	920
Mrs. Paul's Select Cuts:				
Buffalo Shrimp	20	320	15	970
Cheese & Crab Poppers	4	320	16	800
Deviled Crab Cakes	1	180	10	440
Fried Clams	23	320	15	720
Fried Scallops	13	220	7	440
Mini Crab Cakes	6	220	12	480
Stuff Shrimp	3	290	13	720
Singleton:				
Popcorn Scallops	14	180	9	540
Shrimp Poppers	15	200	7	560
Van de Kamp's:				
Crab Cakes	1	170	9	460
Crunchy Popcorn Shrimp	20	270	12	850
Crunchy Butterfly Shrimp	7	300	15	610
Fried Clams	23	320	15	720

Macaroni and Cheese

Ask any child nutrition expert which food most children like best and they will report *macaroni and cheese*! It is obviously a food preference that follows into adult years. Every major brand of frozen entrée offers macaroni and cheese as a complete meal. In addition, there is an expanding array of packaged mixes to select for easy preparation in the microwave or saucepan.

Keeping the portion to 1 cup is essential to control sodium levels in the meal. Watch the nutrition label to select a brand with reduced fat content.

Brand	Serving Size	Calories	Fat (g)	Sodium (mg)	Carbohy-drates (g)
	Frozen Meals				
Stouffer's:					
Lean Cuisine					
Macaroni & Cheese	1 pkg. (283 g)	290	7	630	41
Macaroni & Cheese	1 cup (225 g)				
	(½ pkg.)	320	16	990	31
Weight Watchers:					
Smart Ones Traditional					
Macaroni and Cheese	1 pkg. (283 g)	240	3	800	45
	Dry Mixes				
Kraft:					
Deluxe Original Macaroni & Cheese	1 cup	320	10	870	44
Light Deluxe Macaroni & Cheese	1 cup	290	5	810	48
Macaroni & Cheese	1 cup	260	19	750	48
Velveeta Shells and Cheese	1 cup	360	13	960	46

Skillet Meals

Skillet meals and stir fry have never been easier than they are today. The plastic bags in the frozen food case that previously were used for vegetables and fruits now contain a complete meal that only requires cooking. Most of these are ready to eat in less than 10 minutes!

Although frozen skillet meals may not taste as good as homemade meals, even the fastest chef can't produce beef teriyaki and rice or Romano herb chicken with roasted potatoes in 10 minutes. Speed comes at a price, though. These dishes cost more than making the same dish from scratch, and the portion sizes listed in the nutrition label will not satisfy most consumers. Adding a salad, extra vegetable, or slice of toast may satisfy some, but many will probably reach for a second portion, sending the sodium levels for the meal into overdrive.

Brand	Serving Size	Calories	Fat (g)	Sodium (mg)
Birds Eye Chicken Voila!:				
Alfredo Chicken	1 cup	250	9	710
Garden Herb Chicken	1 cup	320	15	560
Garlic Chicken	1 cup	260	11	540
Pesto Chicken	1 cup	250	9	720
Romano Herb Chicken w/				
Roasted Potatoes	1 cup	220	7	710
Teriyaki	1 cup	230	9	660
Three Cheese Chicken	1 cup	240	9	630
Birds Eye Shrimp Voila!:				
Garlic Shrimp	1 cup	230	9	590
Birds Eye Steak Voila!:				
Beef Sirloin Steak & Garlic Potatoes	1 cup	240	9	650
Chef's Choice:				
Chicken Marinara	1 cup	230	4	740
Chicken Santa Fe	1 cup	230	3	1,090
Chicken Stir Fry	1 cup	190	2	1,130
Shrimp Fried Rice	1 cup	220	2	940

Continued overleaf

Brand	Serving Size	Calories	Fat (g)	Sodium (mg)
Shrimp Linguini	1 cup	180	1	720
Shrimp Stir Fry	1 cup	140	1	900
Steak Ranchero	1 cup	230	4	990
Teriyaki Beef Stir Fry	1 cup	170	3	820
Stouffer's Lean Cuisine Skillet Sensations:				
Beef Teriyaki & Rice	1½ cups	280	3	700
Cheddar Beef	1½ cups	600	29	1,340
Chicken Alfredo	1½ cups	450	16	910
Chicken Oriental	1½ cups	280	3	790
Chicken Primavera	1½ cups	320	5	790
Herb Chicken & Roasted Potatoes	1½ cups	270	5	790
Homestyle Beef	1½ cups	360	11	1,090
Homestyle Chicken	1½ cups	350	9	1,120
Roasted Turkey	1½ cups	220	2	790
Teriyaki Chicken	1½ cups	340	3	1,350
Trader Joe's:				
Chicken, Vegetables & Herb Roasted Potatoes	1 cup	140	3	430

Pizza

Twenty-five years ago pizza was considered a snack. Today, it is a main course and the most popular home-delivered food in North America. Not everyone, however, has the option or desire to call for pizza delivery, so keeping a frozen supply can ensure a tasty meal.

Food technology has even produced a means of making single-serving pizzas in the microwave oven. A disk is supplied in each package that helps firm the crust. These same pizzas can be made in a conventional or toaster oven as well. Overcooking in the microwave and conventional oven results in significant nutritional losses.

One rule of thumb to remember in selecting prepared pizzas: the more cheese and cured meats (i.e., pepperoni, sausage), the higher the sodium and fat levels. Most of the major brands come very close or exceed the 1,000-milligram per serving of sodium recommended per meal.

Brand	Serving Size (g)	Calories	Fat (g)	Sodium (mg)	Carbohy-drates (g)
Amy's Organic Crust and Tomatoes:					
Soy Cheese Pizza	123	280	11	490	37
Celeste Pizza for One:					
Cheese	170	420	20	840	43
Pepperoni	170	470	27	1,060	43
Suprema	221	530	29	1,290	48
DiGiorno:					
Pepperoni	148	390	17	1,080	41
Spicy Chicken Supreme	160	340	11	950	42
Red Barron:					
4 Cheese	153	420	22	800	37
Deep Dish Pepperoni Singles	170	480	27	890	42
Pepperoni	154	440	25	1,020	37
Stouffer's French Bread Pizza:					
Extra Cheese	167	400	16	950	49
Pepperoni	159	390	16	840	48
Tombstone:					
Extra Cheese	145	350	15	640	37
Pepperoni	152	410	22	870	37
Supreme	130	330	17	670	29
Totino's Crisp Crust:					
Cheese	139	320	14	620	34
Pepperoni	145	380	21	910	34
Sausage	153	380	20	880	35
Supreme	155	390	21	900	35
Wolfgang Puck's:					
Four Cheese	130	360	15	530	40
Pepperoni & Mushroom	155	390	15	690	43

Cheese

The ultimate in quick, convenience protein foods is cheese. The selection, though, can be daunting to someone who wants to pick up a healthy choice for sandwiches, salads, and snacking.

Taste buds vary. Some people can't eat a bagel without cream cheese. Others want extra cheese on a pizza. Still others like the spicy cheeses for sprinkling on tacos. One tip to remember in buying cheese is that a significant percentage of the calories comes from fat unless a low-fat selection is made.

For convenience, grated or shredded cheeses are available. In the past, most cheese slices were cut from a block. Today, individually wrapped slices ensure a perfect slice each time. Of course, in most cases, the processing to make these products adds significantly to the sodium content.

Brand	Serving Size	Calories	Fat (g)	Sodium (mg)
	Cheese Products			
Healthy Choice:				
Fancy Cheddar Shreds	¼ cup	50	2	220
Fancy Mozzarella Shreds	¼ cup	50	2	220
Fat-Free Cream Cheese	2 tbsp.	25	0	200
Singles: American,				
Sharp, Cheddar, Swiss	1 slice	40	1	200
Kraft Natural Cheeses:				
Cheddar	1 oz.	120	10	180
Cheddar, Fat-Free	1 oz.	45	0	200
Cheddar, Mild	1 oz.	90	6	240
Colby	1 oz.	110	9	180
Colby, Reduced Fat	1 oz.	80	6	220
Havarti	1 oz.	120	11	240
Monterey Jack	1 oz.	80	6	240
Mozzarella, Fat-Free	1 oz.	45	0	280
Mozzarella, Shredded	⅓ cup	90	6	220
Swiss, Baby	1 oz.	110	9	110

Brand	Serving Size	Calories	Fat (g)	Sodium (mg)
Kraft Processed Cheeses:				
American, 2% Singles	1 slice	50	3	320
American Deluxe Slices	1 slice	110	9	460
American, Free Singles	1 slice	30	0	300
Cheez Whiz	2 tbsp.	90	7	540
Mozzarella, Free Singles	1 slice	30	0	270
Velveeta	1 oz.	90	6	420
Velveeta Light	1 oz.	60	3	440
Kraft Philadelphia Cream Cheese				
(tub = 2 tablespoons/serving):				
Tub & Block, ⅓ Less Fat	1 oz.	70	6	120
Tub & Block, Free	1 oz.	30	0	140
Tub & Block, Regular	1 oz.	100	10	90
Sargento:				
Colby, Deli Style	1 slice	80	7	130
Crumbled Blue Cheese	¼ cup	100	8	360
Light Ricotta	¼ cup	60	3	55
Muenster, Deli Style	1 slice	80	6	140
Ricotta	¼ cup	90	6	75
Shredded Light Mozzarella	¼ cup	70	4	200
Shredded Light Reduced Fat Taco Cheese	¼ cup	70	5	240
String Cheese	1 piece	70	5	170

Vegetarian Meal Choices

Those wanting vegetarian meal choices don't have to spend hours in the kitchen cooking lentils and beans. The frozen meals come with many flavorings with international taste appeal.

Soy products from hot dogs to deli slices and sausage links are available for the vegetarian wanting the convenience of prepared foods.

Continued overleaf

Brand	Serving Size	Calories	Fat (g)	Sodium (mg)
Frozen Meals				
Cascadian Farm Meals for a Small Planet:				
Aztec	1½ cups	290	4	550
Cajun	1½ cups	290	3	600
Indian	1½ cups	340	5	610
Mediterranean	1½ cups	230	7	440
Moroccan	1½ cups	310	5	410
Szechuan	1½ cups	340	9	680
Birds Eye Pasta Secrets:				
Italian Pesto	1 cup	240	9	700
Primavera	1 cup	230	10	430
Ranch	1 cup	300	15	460
Zesty Garlic	1 cup	240	10	310
Trader Joes:				
Berijani Curried Rice Dish	1 cup	170	0	650
Potato Medley	1 cup	120	3	640
Frozen Entrées				
Veggie Patch:				
Chick'n Veggie Cutlets	1 cutlet	140	5	410
Veggie Rounds	1 veggie round	90	4	280
Bowl Meals				
Yves Veggie Cuisine:				
Veggie Country Stew	1 container	170	0	1,020
Veggie Lasagna	1 container	300	3	650

Brand	Serving Size	Calories	Fat (g)	Sodium (mg)
"Hot Dogs"				
Lightlife:				
Smart Deli Jumbo	2½ oz.	80	0	590
Smart Dogs	1½ oz.	50	0	170
Wonderdogs	1½ oz.	60	1	170
Loma Linda:				
Big Franks	2 oz.	110	7	240
Linketts	1 oz.	70	5	160
Low-Fat Big Franks	2 oz.	80	3	220
Morningstar Farms:				
Veggie Dogs	2 oz.	80	1	580
Nasoya:				
New Menu Veggie Dog	1½ oz.	50	0	170
Soy Boy:				
Leaner Wieners	1½ oz.	60	0	140
Worthington:				
Leanies	1½ oz.	110	8	430
Low-Fat Veja-Links	1 oz.	40	2	190
Super-Links	1½ oz.	110	8	350
Veja-Links	1 oz.	50	3	190
Yves:				
Hot and Spicy Jumbo Veggie Dogs	2½ oz.	100	0	420
Jumbo Veggie Dogs	2½ oz.	90	0	570
Original Tofu Pups	1½ oz.	60	3	140
Tofu Wieners	1½ oz.	50	1	240
Veggie Chili Dogs	1½ oz.	60	0	300
Veggie Wieners	1½ oz.	60	0	340
"Veggie Burgers" and "Drumsticks"				
Amy's:				
Chicago Veggie Burger	1 patty	100	4	190
Texas BBQ Veggie Burger	1 patty	130	2	270
Veggie Burger	1 patty	130	2	270
Garden Gourmet:				
Vegetarian Burger	1 patty	100	4	440
Vegetarian Drumsticks	1	90	4	400
Vegetarian Veggie-Pattie	1 patty	90	4	430

Continued overleaf

Brand	Serving Size	Calories	Fat (g)	Sodium (mg)
Gardenburger:				
Hamburger Style	1 patty	90	1	320
Original Veggie	1 patty	130	3	290
Roasted Garlic	1 patty	90	1	200
Savory Mushroom	1 patty	120	2	370
Morningstar Farms (Worthington Foods):				
Chik Patties	1 patty	150	6	570
Garden Veggie Patties	1 patty	100	3	350
Harvest Burgers	1 patty	140	4	370
Whole Foods:				
Meat Free Garlic Burger	1 patty	80	1	240
Meat Free Gourmet Burger	1 patty	100	2	290
Meat Free Vegan Burger	1 patty	80	0	270

"Sausage"

Brand	Serving Size	Calories	Fat (g)	Sodium (mg)
Cedar Lake:				
Breakfast Sausage	2 links (2½ oz.)	180	10	550
Garden Sausage	1 patty (2½ oz.)	140	3	460
Lightlife:				
Breakfast Lean Links	2 links (2½ oz.)	120	6	260
Gimme Lean! Sausage	2 oz.	70	0	290
Italian Lean Links	1 link (1½ oz.)	60	2	160
Lightsausages	2 patties (2½ oz.)	80	0	340
Loma Linda:				
Little Links	2 links (1½ oz.)	90	6	230
Morningstar Farms:				
Breakfast Links	2 links (1½ oz.)	60	3	340
Breakfast Patties	1 patty (1½ oz.)	70	3	270
Natural Touch:				
Vegan Sausage Crumbles	2 oz.	60	0	300
Worthington:				
Posage Links	2 links (2½ oz.)	60	3	340
Posage Patties	1 patty (2½ oz.)	80	3	300
Yves:				
Veggie Breakfast Links	2 links (2 oz.)	70	0	360

Brand	Serving Size	Calories	Fat (g)	Sodium (mg)
"Bacon"				
Lightlife Fakin' Bacon				
Smokey Tempeh Strips	1 strip (⅔ oz.)	30	1	80
Morningstar Farms Breakfast Strips	2 strips (½ oz.)	60	5	220
Worthington Stripples	2 strips (½ oz.)	60	5	220
Yves Canadian Veggie Bacon	3 slices (2 oz.)	80	0	490
"Deli Slices"				
Lightlife Smart Deli:				
Country Ham	4 slices (2 oz.)	70	0	400
Foney Baloney	4 slices (2 oz.)	80	3	320
Old World Bologna	4 slices (2 oz.)	70	0	400
Roast Turkey	4 slices (2 oz.)	50	0	390
Three Peppercorn	4 slices (2 oz.)	60	0	400
Tofurky Deli Slices:				
Hickory Smoked	4 slices (2 oz.)	160	2	440
Original	4 slices (2 oz.)	160	2	380
Vegi-Deli Slice of Life:				
Chicken	4 slices (2 oz.)	100	2	340
Pepperoni	10 slices (2 oz.)	140	3	320
Salami	4 slices (2 oz.)	130	3	340
Turkey	4 slices (2 oz.)	110	3	370
White Wave:				
Chicken-Style Sandwich	2 slices (2 oz.)	80	0	260
Pastrami-Style Sandwich	2 slices (2 oz.)	90	0	270
Turkey-Style Sandwich	2 slices (2 oz.)	80	0	400
Worthington Meatless:				
Bolono	3 slices (2 oz.)	80	4	720
Chicken	2 slices (2 oz.)	80	5	370
Corned Beef	4 slices (2 oz.)	140	9	520
Salami	3 slices (2 oz.)	130	8	930
Smoked Beef	6 slices (2 oz.)	120	6	730
Smoked Turkey	3 slices (2 oz.)	140	10	620
Wham	2 slices (2 oz.)	80	5	430
Yves:				
Deli Slices	4 slices (2 oz.)	70	0	530
Veggie Pepperoni	4 slices (2 oz.)	80	0	380

Meal Accompaniments

Every day the dilemma of what to make with the chicken breast and broccoli creates anxiety for the cook. Side dishes or accompaniments don't have to be limited to quick rice, noodles, or potatoes baked in the microwave. Review this list of meal accompaniments to add more variety to your menus. Watch out for ones with lots of fat and sodium.

Brand	Serving Size	Calories	Fat (g)	Sodium (mg)
Potatoes				
French fries:				
Cascadian Farm Oven Fries	30	220	7	15
McDonald's French Fries	Large	450	22	290
Ore-Ida Cottage Fries	23	220	7	35
Ore-Ida Country Style Steak Fries	13	180	6	480
Ore-Ida Golden Crinkles	23	230	6	35
Ore-Ida Golden Fries	25	200	7	40
Ore-Ida Oven Roast	17	150	4	520
Ore-Ida Seasoned Plus Potato Wedges	8	220	8	820
Ore-Ida Shoestrings	63	250	8	35
Ore-Ida Steak Fries	12	180	5	35
Ore-Ida Texas Crispers!	13	250	12	530
Hash browns and home fries:				
Bob Evan's Home Fries, Original	1 cup	190	7	860
Cascadian Farm Organic Hash Browns	1⅔ cups	180	7	35
Fresh from the Start Ready-to-Cook Home-Fried Potatoes	1 cup	100	0	26
McDonald's Hash Browns	1 order	130	8	330
Ore-Ida Country Style Hash Browns	2 cups	190	7	25
Ore-Ida Microwave Hash Browns	4 oz. pkg.	110	6	150
Ore-Ida Potatoes O'Brien	1¼ cups	160	7	40
Mashed:				
Betty Crocker Potato Buds	⅔ cup	160	8	460
Ore-Ida Mashed Potatoes (2% milk)	⅔ cup	150	4	240

Brand	Serving Size	Calories	Fat (g)	Sodium (mg)
Others:				
Fresh from the Start Ready to Cook				
Red Bliss Potatoes	1 cup	100	0	26
Ore-Ida Tater Tots	15	270	13	570
Ore-Ida Topped Baked Potatoes,				
Broccoli & Cheese	½ potato	160	4	480
Stouffer's Potatoes Au Gratin	½ cup	130	6	590
Stouffer's Scalloped Potatoes	½ cup	180	8	540
Trader Joe's Herb-Roasted Potatoes	1 cup	110	0	210

Stuffing Mixes

Brand	Serving Size	Calories	Fat (g)	Sodium (mg)
Kraft Stove Top Oven Classics:				
Lemon Chicken Bake	⅙ box	220	1	500
Traditional Roast Chicken Bake	⅙ box	190	3	870

Rice and Pasta Mixes

Brand	Serving Size	Calories	Fat (g)	Sodium (mg)
Betty Crocker:				
Cheddar & Broccoli Rice	1 cup	240	6	880
Creamy Garlic & Herb Rotini	1 cup	240	5	720
Creamy Herb Risotto Rice	1 cup	270	7	760
Garlic Alfredo Fettuccine Pasta	1 cup	220	3	700
Lipton:				
Noodles & Sauce Alfredo Broccoli	1 cup	260	7	870
Noodles & Sauce Chicken Broccoli	1 cup	230	4	740
Pasta & Sauce 3 Cheese Rotini	1 cup	240	5	870
Rice-a-Roni:				
Chicken Flavor	1 cup	310	1	1,000
Chicken and Broccoli	1 cup	230	1	950
Pasta Roni Angel Hair Pasta w/				
Parmesan Cheese	1 cup	210	5	740
Pasta Roni White Cheddar &				
Broccoli with Rigatoni	1 cup	210	5	650
Success Rice:				
Broccoli & Cheese Mix	½ cup	210	4.5	840
Classic Chicken Mix	½ cup	150	1	720
Uncle Ben's:				
Country Inn Broccoli Rice Au Gratin	1 cup	200	2	790
Country Inn Chicken & Vegetable	1 cup	190	2	580

Continued overleaf

Brand	Serving Size	Calories	Fat (g)	Sodium (mg)
Frozen Vegetable Blends				
Birds Eye:				
Creamed Spinach	½ cup	100	7	660
Gold & White Corn Blend	½ cup	60	1	330
Radiatore Pasta & Vegetables	1 cup	200	8	430
Roasted Potatoes & Broccoli	⅔ cup	100	4	470
Cascadian Farm:				
Broccoli w/Cheddar Cheese Sauce	½ cup	60	3	290
French Green Bean Casserole (Organic)	¾ cup	90	5	360
French Green Beans w/Toasted Almonds	¾ cup	70	3	115
Honey Glazed Baby Carrots	1 cup	60	0	160
Peas & Pearl Onions	¾ cup	60	0	130
Potatoes Au Gratin	⅔ cup	110	4	290
Winter Squash	½ cup	50	0	5
Goya:				
Ripe Plantains	4 pieces	210	8	0
Green Giant:				
Alfredo Vegetables	¾ cup	80	3	450
Baby Brussels Sprouts & Butter	½ cup	60	2	270
Broccoli, Cauliflower, Carrots & Cheese	⅔ cup	80	3	560
Primavera Pasta	1 pkg.	300	10	930
Southwest Style Corn & Roasted Red Peppers	¾ cup	90	1	130
Uncle Ben's:				
Black Bean and Vegetable	1 bowl		4	850
Rice Bowl Southwest Style	1 bowl		4	850

Pasta Sauces

Pasta is an economical and convenient meal that only requires cooking the pasta and selecting an appropriate sauce. The number of pasta sauces available rival the shapes and sizes of pasta, so no two pasta meals need to be alike.

Pasta sauces can be purchased in cans, jars, or plastic containers (from the refrigerated section of the supermarket). Dried sauce mixes are available, but they don't seem to command the consumer's attention like the ready-to-use choices.

Prepared sauces can be high in fat and sodium, so it is prudent to either limit portion sizes or select a brand that has been modified to meet nutritional guidelines.

Brand	Variety	Serving Size	Calories	Fat (g)	Sodium (mg)	Carbohy-drates (g)
Balsamic	Traditional	½ cup	80	3	510	14
Barilla	Marinara	½ cup	70	2	430	11
	Pesto	¼ cup	280	28	810	3
Butoni	Garden Vegetable	½ cup	60	2	260	9
	Marinara	½ cup	80	3	440	14
Chef Boyardee	Spaghetti Sauce w/Meat	½ cup	90	2	819	15
Classico	Alfredo	¼ cup	110	10	480	3
	Florentine Spinach & Cheese	½ cup	80	4	490	8
	Spicy Tomato & Pesto	½ cup	90	5	530	9
	Tomato & Basil	½ cup	50	1	390	9
Contadina	Alfredo	¼ cup	180	16	270	5
(Refrigerated)	Alfredo Light	¼ cup	80	5	330	5
	Marinara	½ cup	80	4	550	9
	Pesto	¼ cup	290	24	580	12
	Pesto Reduced Fat	¼ cup	230	18	560	11
Healthy Choice	Chunky Vegetable Primavera	½ cup	45	0	390	10
	Mushroom Alfredo	¼ cup	45	3	430	3
	Traditional	½ cup	50	0	390	11
Hunt's	Four Cheese	½ cup	50	1	600	9
	Light Traditional	½ cup	40	0	420	9
	Traditional	½ cup	60	1	640	11
Newman's Own	Five Cheese	½ cup	90	3	510	14
	Venetian Marinara	½ cup	60	2	590	9
Prego	Garden Combination	½ cup	100	2	480	19

Continued overleaf

Brand	Variety	Serving Size	Calories	Fat (g)	Sodium (mg)	Carbohy- drates (g)
	Italian Sausage & Garlic	½ cup	120	5	500	16
	Ricotta Parmesan	½ cup	120	3	500	20
	Three Cheese	½ cup	100	2	460	18
Progresso	Alfredo	½ cup	200	15	850	7
	White Clam	½ cup	140	10	510	5

Seasoned Coating Mixes for Main Dishes

Glazing, breading, or seasoning chicken, pork, or seafood is easy when you pick up a coating mix that comes complete with spices, herbs, and flour and is guaranteed to please everyone's palate. Gone are the days when the busy consumer seasoned chicken with a canned soup mix or salad dressing blend. These products supply all the flavoring ingredients in one box.

Of course, you have to remember to buy the main dish—chicken, pork chops, or fish—and plan a meal accompaniment plus salad to make a complete menu.

Brand	Serving Size	Calories	Fat (g)	Sodium (mg)
Kraft Oven Fry:				
Extra Crispy Chicken	Coating on 1 piece	60	1	420
Extra Crispy Pork	About ½ oz. coating on 1 chop	60	2	340
Fish Fry	Coating on 1 piece	45	1	290
Kraft Shake 'n Bake glazes:				
Classic Italian (Chicken or Pork)	Coating on 1 piece	40	1	280
Tangy Honey (Chicken or Pork)	Coating on 1 piece	45	1	300
Lipton Recipe Secrets:				
Garlic Mushroom	1½ tbsp. (¼ oz.)	20	0	530
Onion	1 tbsp. (¼ oz.)	20	0	620

Baking Mixes

When the baking urge hits, how do you decide which mix to select in the supermarket? A general rule of thumb for cakes is to forget pineapple upside-down cake, carrot cake, and German chocolate cake. As this comparison illustrates, the angel food cake that was allowed on the diabetic meal plan isn't much lower in carbohydrate content than some chocolate or white cakes. When it comes to cakes, the frosting is the culprit. The carbohydrates and fat in frosting add up very quickly. Two tablespoons of frosting does not go very far in covering a serving of cake.

Home-baked cookies and brownies are another option. They usually have about the same calories and carbohydrates as a serving of cake and don't need frosting to be considered "complete."

Brand	Variety	Serving Size	Calories	Fat (g)	Carbohy-drates (g)
		Cake Mixes			
Betty Crocker	Angel Food				
	One-Step White	½ cake	140	0	32
	Butter Pecan	½ cake	250	11	34
	Carrot	⅒ cake	320	15	42
	Devil's Food, Reduced Fat (Sweet Rewards)	½ cake	200	5	36
	Double Chocolate Swirl	½ cake	250	11	35
	Golden Vanilla	½ cake	280	14	35
	Lemon	½ cake	280	14	35
	Pineapple Upside-Down Cake plus Topping	⅙ cake	400	15	63
	White, Reduced Fat (Sweet Rewards)	½ cake	190	4	36
Duncan Hines	Angel Food	½ cake	140	0	31
	Butter Golden	½ cake	320	16	42
	Lemon Supreme	½ cake	250	11	36
	White	½ cake	190	6	34

Continued overleaf

Brand	Variety	Serving Size	Calories	Fat (g)	Carbohy-drates (g)
Pillsbury	Angel Food	½ cake	140	0	31
	Carrot	½ cake	250	11	34
	Devil's Food	½ cake	270	14	33
	German Chocolate	½ cake	230	9	34
	White	½ cake	270	10	41

Frosting (Ready to Use)

Brand	Variety	Serving Size	Calories	Fat (g)	Carbohy-drates (g)
Betty Crocker	Cherry	2 tbsp.	140	5	24
	Chocolate, Reduced Fat	2 tbsp.	120	3	24
	Coconut Pecan	2 tbsp.	140	8	17
	Dark Chocolate	2 tbsp.	150	6	22
	Sour Cream White	2 tbsp.	150	6	25
	Vanilla, Reduced Fat	2 tbsp.	120	2	26
Duncan Hines	Chocolate	2 tbsp.	130	5	20
	Vanilla	2 tbsp.	140	5	22
Pillsbury	Coconut Pecan	2 tbsp.	160	10	17
	Lemon Creme	2 tbsp.	150	6	24
	Milk Chocolate	2 tbsp.	140	6	21
	Vanilla	2 tbsp.	150	6	23

Cookie and Brownie Mixes

Brand	Variety	Serving Size	Calories	Fat (g)	Carbohy-drates (g)
Betty Crocker	Brownie, Stir 'n Bake w/Mini Kisses	⅛ batch	220	8	35
	Chocolate Chip	2 cookies	170	8	21
	Date Bars	½ batch	150	6	23
	Double Chocolate Chunk	2 cookies	150	6	21
	Fudge Brownie	⅟₂₀ batch	170	7	23
	Low-Fat Fudge Brownie	⅟₁₈ batch	130	3	27
	Oatmeal Chocolate Chip	2 cookies	160	7	21
	Peanut Butter	2 cookies	160	8	20
	Sunkist Lemon Bars	⅟₁₆ batch	140	5	24
Duncan Hines	Chewy Fudge Brownie	½ batch	160	7	25
	Mississippi Mud Brownie	⅟₂₀ batch	160	6	27
Pillsbury	Chocolate Chunk Brownie	⅟₁₆ batch	160	7	22
	Lemon Cheesecake Bars	⅟₂₄ batch	190	10	22
	M&M's Bars	⅟₁₈ batch	170	6	27
	Walnut Brownie	½ batch	190	10	24

Brand	Variety	Serving Size	Calories	Fat (g)	Carbohy-drates (g)
		Refrigerated Cookie Dough			
Nestlé	Brownies	½ pkg.	180	7	26
	Chocolate Chip	1	110	5	16
	Sugar Cookies	1	120	5	18
Pillsbury	Chocolate Chip	1 oz.	140	7	17
	Peanut Butter	1 oz.	130	6	16
Private	Chocolate Chunk	1	120	6	16
Selection	Oatmeal Raisin	1	110	5	16
		Muffin Mixes			
Betty Crocker	Apple Cinnamon	1	170	7	23
	Banana Nut	1	170	7	22
Jiffy	Banana Nut	1	180	7[a]	25
	Blueberry	1	190	7[a]	28
	Corn	1	180	6[a]	28
Martha White	Blueberry	1	150	2	31
Low-Fat	Honey Bran	1	200	7[a]	25
Washington	Blueberry	1	170	6[a]	29
Raga	Carrot and Spice	1	170	6[a]	27

[a]Calculated value based on package ingredients.

Cookies

In the olden days of diabetic meal planning, there were graham crackers, vanilla wafers, more graham crackers, and more vanilla wafers. Today, there are many more choices with about the same sugar content. Those wanting low-fat cookies will find several selections available as well.

Cookies are grouped by type for easier comparison. The graham cracker section will be a revelation to many who have thought that these snacks were low in sugar. "Graham flour" is a whole wheat flour by definition, but most of the varieties available contain less than 10 percent whole wheat flour; so much for the fiber and extra nutrition story on graham crackers.

Cookie/Cracker	Variety	Serving Size	Calories	Fat (g)	Sugar (g)
Chocolate chip	Entenmann's Light Chocolate Chip	2	120	4	13
	Nabisco Chips Ahoy	3	160	8	10
	Nabisco Reduced-Fat Chips Ahoy	3	140	5	10
	Pepperidge Farm Reduced-Fat Chocolate Chunk	1	110	5	8
	SnackWell's Chocolate Chip	13	130	4	10
	SnackWell's Double Chocolate Chip	13	130	4	10
Fruit bars	Health Valley Fat-Free Jumbo Fruit	1	80	0	9
	Nabisco Fat-Free Cobblers	1	70	0	10
	Nabisco Fat-Free Fig Newtons	2	100	0	14
	Nabisco Fig Newtons	2	110	3	14
	Newman's Own Organics Fig Newtons	2	120	0	15
	Weight Watchers Fig Bars	1	70	0	9
Graham crackers	Keebler Graham Selects	8	150	6	8
	Keebler Low-Fat Graham Selects	8	120	2	9
	Keebler Reduced-Fat Deluxe Grahams	3	120	5	11
	Nabisco Honey Maid	8	120	3	8
	Nabisco Low-Fat Honey Maid	8	110	2	9
Oatmeal	Archway Fat-Free Oatmeal Raisin	1	110	0	14
	Archway Oatmeal	1	110	4	8
	Entenmann's Light Oatmeal Raisin	2	100	0	14
	Pepperidge Farm Fat-Free Iced Oatmeal Raisin	2	120	0	12
	Pepperidge Farm Oatmeal Raisin	1	110	4	9
	SnackWell's Oatmeal Raisin	2	120	3	10
Sandwich style	Nabisco Oreo	3	160	7	13
	Nabisco Reduced-Fat Oreo	3	130	4	14
	SnackWell's Creme Sandwich	2	110	3	10
	Sunshine Hydrox	3	150	7	11
	Sunshine Reduced-Fat Hydrox	3	140	5	13
	Weight Watchers Vanilla Sandwich	3	140	3	10
Wafers	Archway Ginger Snaps	5	150	5	11
	Archway Reduced-Fat Ginger Snaps	5	140	4	12
	Keebler Reduced-Fat Vanilla Wafers	9	130	4	11
	Nabisco Nilla Wafers	9	140	5	12

Cookie/Cracker	Variety	Serving Size	Calories	Fat (g)	Sugar (g)
	Nabisco Old Fashioned Ginger Snaps	4	120	3	9
	Nabisco Reduced-Fat Nilla Wafers	9	120	2	12
Other varieties	Archway Fat-Free Devil's Food	1	70	0	8
	Archway Old-Fashioned Molasses	1	100	3	10
	Archway Sugar Cookies	1	10	3	7
	Keebler Reduced-Fat Pecan Sandies	2	140	6	6
	Nabisco Barnum's Animals	10	140	4	7
	Nabisco Lorna Doone	4	140	7	6
	Pepperidge Farm Milano	3	180	10	11
	SnackWell's Devil's Food	2	100	0	14

Sweets and Treats

Desserts are desserts, a treat that needs to be considered in that frame of mind. Cookies, cakes, pies, and pastries may say "fat-free" on the label, but they seldom have a significant reduction in calories from traditional desserts. Nuts, dried fruits, and vegetable oils may be healthier than sugar and honey or butter but they are still highly caloric. Many frozen fruit bars have sugar added to them, but they are a good nonfat dessert. Ice creams, especially the premium kinds, are loaded with fat, but a few decadent desserts for a special occasion can be worked into any meal plan. Moderation is the key.

One of the first questions that a diabetes educator is asked when explaining the meal plan is, "Does diabetes mean I can never eat a Twinkie or a candy bar again?" For some people, that would be no problem; for others, that seems devastating. Although some foods (i.e., Dairy Queen medium chocolate shake or McDonald's McFlurry) are not recommended, eating a Reese's Peanut Butter Cup or Milky Way Lite could possibly be planned into the daily regime.

Comparing these selections may help you make better choices for sweets and treats.

Treat	Variety	Serving Size	Calories	Fat (g)	Sugar (g)
Candy	3 Musketeers	1 2.4 oz.	260	8	40
	Butterfinger	1 2.1 oz.	270	11	29
	Junior Mints	1 1.6 oz. box	180	3	37
	Kit Kat	1 1.5 oz. pkg.	220	11	21
	M&Ms	1 1.7 oz. pkg.	240	10	31
	Milky Way	1 2.1 oz.	270	10	35
	Milky Way Lite	1 1.6 oz.	170	5	24
	Reese's Peanut Butter Cups	2 1.6 oz.	250	14	21
	Skittles	1 2 oz. pkg.	240	3	45
	Snickers	1 2.1 oz.	280	14	29
	Twizzlers Strawberry Twists	10 2.5 oz.	230	1	26
Doughnuts	Entenmann's Glazed 50% Less Fat	1	220	6	27
	Entenmann's Rich-Frosted Donuts	1	280	19	15
	Hostess Frosted Donettes	3	200	12	13
	Hostess Powdered Donettes	3	180	9	10
	Krispy Kreme Fudge Iced Creme Filled	1 3 oz.	340	18	22
	Krispy Kreme Glazed Raspberry Filled	1 3 oz.	270	12	20
	Krispy Kreme Original Glazed	1	210	12	13
Ice cream & yogurt	Baskin Robbins Chocolate Ice Cream	1 cup	300	18	32
	Breyers Fat-Free Vanilla Ice Cream	1 cup	220	0	42
	Breyers Natural Vanilla Ice Cream	1 cup	300	18	30
	Cascade Glacier Oregon Cherry Indulgence	1 cup	380	22	40
	Cascade Glacier Triple Chocolate Aftershock	1 cup	400	26	38
	Dairy Queen Chocolate Malt (medium)	20 oz.	880	22	131
	Dairy Queen Chocolate Shake (medium)	19 oz.	770	20	113
	Dairy Queen Vanilla Cone (large)	20 oz.	410	12	49
	Fruit a Freeze Banana Chocolate-Dipped Fruit Bar	1	170	9	22
	Fruit a Freeze Coconut Chocolate-Dipped Fruit Bar	1	210	13	23

Treat	Variety	Serving Size	Calories	Fat (g)	Sugar (g)
	Fruit a Freeze Strawberry Banana Energy Smoothie Bar	1	120	3	21
	Häagen-Dazs Chocolate Chocolate Chip Ice Cream	1 cup	600	40	48
	Häagen-Dazs Chocolate Ice Cream	1 cup	540	36	42
	Häagen-Dazs Low-Fat Chocolate Ice Cream	1 cup	340	5	30
	McDonald's Hot Fudge Sundae	1 cup	340	12	47
	McDonald's McFlurry	20 oz.	610	22	75
	McDonald's Vanilla Shake	6.5 oz.	480	13	71
	Wendy's Frosty	9 oz.	540	14	70
Muffins	Entenmann's Light Blueberry	1	120	0	15
	Entenmann's Little Bites Blueberry Mini-Muffins	4	190	8	16
	Healthy Valley Fat-Free Healthy Scones	1	180	0	18
	Hostess Cream Cheese Hearty	1 6 oz.	620	33	41
	Hostess Oat Bran	1	160	8	9
	Sara Lee Blueberry	1	220	11	12
	Weight Watchers Smart Ones	1	170	1	15
Pastries	Entenmann's Cinnamon Swirl Buns	1 3 oz.	300	13	19
	Entenmann's Light Cinnamon Buns	1 2 oz.	160	3	17
	Hostess Cup Cakes	1 2 oz.	180	6	17
	Hostess Lights Low-Fat Cupcakes	1 1.5 oz.	140	2	19
	Hostess Lights Low-Fat Twinkies	1 1.5 oz.	130	2	16
	Hostess Twinkies	1 1.5 oz.	150	5	14
	Little Debbie Apple Streusel Coffee Cakes	2 2 oz.	230	7	23
	Little Debbie Fudge Brownies	1 1.5 oz.	310	15	28
	McDonald's Cheese Danish	1 3.5 oz.	410	22	26
	Mrs. Fields Double-Fudge Brownie	1 3 oz.	420	25	47
	Nabisco Frosted Toastettes, Brown Sugar Cinnamon	1 tart	190	8	35
	Nabisco Frosted Toastettes Strawberry	1 tart	190	8	35
	Philadelphia Chocolate Chip Cheesecake Snack Bar	1	200	13	17
	Philadelphia Classic Cheesecake Snack Bar	1	200	13	17

Snack Bars

Portability of foods that offer nutrition in a little package is important for many consumers, including people with diabetes. Food bars can be anything from a quick snack to a meal replacement that tucks into a briefcase, backpack, or purse for quick consumption when time does not allow a traditional meal.

Today's snack bars have been greatly enhanced since the concept of "energy bars" originated for athletes in the mid-1980s. Many contain nutrient levels equivalent to a meal of 200 to 300 calories with 100 percent of the U. S. Recommended Daily Intake of many vitamins and minerals.

These food bars promise guilt-free eating for the granola bar lover or the midafternoon snacker who previously devoured a candy bar. They can be part of a healthy diet if prudence is used in quantity eaten and if adequate hydration accompanies their consumption.

Some bars are designed strictly as a snack item for people with diabetes. These products usually contain a resistant cornstarch (uncooked cornstarch) that is not completely digested so that there is less glucose (sugar) absorbed from the bar. These products can be used as a quick snack or sweet treat without the guilt feelings that may accompany a cookie or candy bar.

Food Bar, Size & Flavor	Calories	Protein (g)	Sodium (mg)	Fat (g)	Carbo-hydrates (g)
[1] Advantage Bar, (Atkins Diet), 60 g					
Chocolate Macadamia Nut	240	18	196	13	2.6
[2] Balance, 50 g					
Honey Peanut, Almond Brownie,					
Chocolate Raspberry Fudge	190	14	140	6	22
[3] Boost Nutritional Energy Bar, 44 g					
Strawberries and Cream,					
Chocolate Crunch	190	5	50	6	30
[4] Breakthru, 60 g					
Cinnamon Crunch, Mocha Fudge,					
Honey Graham, Chocolate Fudge	220	12	160	3	37

Food Bar, Size & Flavor	Calories	Protein (g)	Sodium (mg)	Fat (g)	Carbo-hydrates (g)
[5] Choice for people with diabetes, 35 g					
Peanutty Chocolate Fudge Brownie	140	6	60	4.5	17
[6] CLIF Bar,					
The Natural Energy Bar, 68 g					
Chocolate Chip, Carrot Cake,					
Cookies 'n Cream, Real Berry,					
Apple Cherry, Chocolate Espresso,					
Apricot	250	4	45	3	51
[7] Ensure, 39 g					
[8] Ensure Glucerna Bar	140	5	100	4	24
Honey Graham Crust, Chocolate					
Fudge Brownie	130	6	115	3	21
[9] GeniSoy, 61.5 g					
Chocolate coated	220	14	190	3.5	33
[10] Gluc-o-Bar, 37 g					
Strawberry-Banana, Chocolate,					
Peanut Butter	130	7	105	2	22
[11] Harvest Energy Bar, 65 g					
Chocolate, Strawberry	240	7	80	4	45
[12] Met-RX "engineered nutrition," 100 g					
Extreme Vanilla	320	27	110	2.5	48
[13] Mountain Lift, 60 g					
Peanut Crunch	220	12	180	4.5	33
[14] NiteBite Time-release Glucose Bar, 25 g					
Peanut Butter, Chocolate Fudge	100	3	80	3.5	15
[15] Nutri-Grain Cereal Bar, 37 g					
Raspberry, etc.	140	2	110	3	27
[16] PR Ironman, 56.8 g					
Creamy Peanut	230	16	280	8	23
[17] Power Bar Athletic Energy Bar, 65 g					
Mocha, Apple Cinnamon, Banana,					
Peanut Butter, Chocolate	230	10	90	2.5	45
Protein 21, 53 g					
Fudge Brownie, Cinnamon,					
Golden Almond Crunch	190	21	380	7	10
[18] Prozone, 50 g					
Raspberry Burst, Mango	194	14	90	6	18
[19] Standard Bar, 50 g					
Peanut Butter, etc.	200	12	70	7	24

Continued overleaf

Food Bar, Size & Flavor	Calories	Protein (g)	Sodium (mg)	Fat (g)	Carbo- hydrates (g)
[20] Sweet Rewards Fat-Free, 32 g					
Double Fudge Brownie	100	2	90	0	25
[21] Sweet Success Chocolate Candy Bars, 31 g					
Caramel, Honey, and Nougat	100	1	45	3.5	23
[22] THINK, 56.7 g					
Chocolate Almond, Coconut Raisin, Apple Spice, Chocolate Coated	230	6	42	5	39
[23] Tiger's Milk, 35 g	145	7	70	5	18
[24] Ultimate Protein Bar, 78 g					
Chocolate Peanut Butter Supreme	280	32	50	6	19
[25] York Diet Bar, 49 g	200	9	180	6	28
[26] Zone Perfect, 50 g					
Almond Crunch, Chocolate Almond Fudge	190	14	150	6	20

1 Atkins Nutritionals, Bohemia, NY (product of Canada)
2 BioFoods, Inc., Carpinteria, CA
3 Mead Johnson and Co., Evansville, IN
4 Glenn Foods, Valley Stream, NY
5 Mead Johnson and Co., Evansville, IN
6 KALI's Sport Naturals, Inc., Berkeley, CA
7 Ross Products, Division of Abbott Laboratories, Columbus, OH
8 Ross Products, Division of Abbott Laboratories, Columbus, OH
9 GeniSoy Products Co., Fairfield, CA
10 Amoun Pharmaceutical Company, Westmont, IL
11 Powerbar, Inc., Berkeley, CA
12 Met RX USA, Irvine, CA
13 M L Industries, Chatsworth, CA
14 Medical Foods, Inc., Cambridge, MA
15 Kellogg Company, Battle Creek, MI
16 PR Nutrition, Inc., San Diego, CA
17 Powerfood, Inc., Berkeley, CA
18 NutriBiotic, Lakeport, CA
19 Standard Process, Inc., Palmyra, WI
20 General Mills, Minneapolis, MN
21 Nestlé USA. Nutritional Division, Glendale, CA (product of Mexico)
22 Ph.D. Personal Health Development, Ventura, CA
23 Weider Nutrition Group, Salt Lake City, UT
24 Country Life
25 York Barbell Co., York, PA
26 Eicotech Corp., Marblehead, MA

Chapter 8
Caution:
Restaurant Meals

---

*R*estaurant eating may spell disaster when eating on the run. Some restaurant serving sizes are equivalent to a full day's worth of calories, fat, and protein! Dividing the portion in half when it is delivered to the table may still result in overeating. A study of restaurant meals published by *Tufts University Health and Nutrition Letter*, February 2001, revealed some huge portions. Here are some of the results and suggestions on how to modify the meals.

Applebee's	*Triple Decker Club* = 5 ounces meat, cheese + 5 ounces bread (average sandwich = 2–3 ounces meat, cheese + 2 ounces bread)
	Steakhouse Salad = 7 ounces steak + 1½ ounces cheese (average chicken/beef Caesar = 3–4 ounces meat + ½ ounce cheese)
Bennigan's	*Fried Cheese Sticks* (appetizer) = 5 ounces cheese (enough for a main course)
	Health Club Chicken Platter = 7 ounces chicken + 1½ cups rice (divide into two meals)
Chili's	*Chicken Fajita Quesadillas* = 3 tortillas, 4½ ounces chicken, 2 cups rice (divide into two meals)

Houlihan's	*BBQ, full slab, with French fries* = 15 ounces meat + 70 french fries (enough meat for two entire days + seven servings of french fries!)
Olive Garden	*Chicken Parmesan* = 9 ounces chicken + 1 ounce cheese + 1 plus cup spaghetti + 2 bread sticks (divide into two meals)
	Spaghetti and Meatballs = 3 cups spaghetti + 7 ounces meat + 2 bread sticks (divide into two meals)
TGI Friday's	*Friday's Shrimp* = 4 ounces shrimp + 44 french fries (leave half the fries!)

According to the U. S. Department of Health and Human Services, Americans may be eating better than they did in the 1980s, but diets still need improvement. The new dietary guidelines are not focused specifically on the excesses of restaurant meals, but they certainly apply.

Choosing a diet low in *saturated* fat requires less use of high-fat dairy products and fatty meats. Eating more fish and lean poultry foods such as turkey, Cornish hens, and chicken can make a difference in a daily menu.

Here are two examples to illustrate the difference between a high-saturated-fat menu at a restaurant and a low-saturated-fat menu at home. Notice the total fat and saturated fat differences. The polyunsaturated fat/saturated fat ratio is also important to consider. The high-saturated-fat menu has no meal with a polyunsaturated fat/saturated fat ratio greater than 1, but all meals in the low-saturated-fat menu have a ratio greater than 1.

In Chapter 10, "Fast-Food Comparisons," you will find some choices that are low in fat. Remember them when you are needing a quick meal so that your total fat and saturated fat levels can stay in the healthy range.

High-Saturated-Fat Menu at Restaurant

	Amount	Total Fat (g)	Saturated Fat (g)	Polyunsaturated Fat (g)	Monounsaturated Fat (g)	Saturated Fat Ratio	Cholesterol (mg)
BREAKFAST — Egg McMuffin (1), Orange juice (4 oz.), Milk, whole (8 oz.)							
Breakfast							
Egg McMuffin	1	11	4	1	6		226
Orange juice	4 oz.						
Milk, whole	8 oz.	8	5		3		34
Total		**19**	**9**	**1**	**9**	**0.11**	**260**
LUNCH — Big Mac, Fries (regular), Apple pie							
Lunch							
Big Mac	1	32	10	1.5	21		103
Fries, regular	1	17	7	1.0	9		12
Apple pie	1	15	5	1.0	9		12
Total		**64**	**22**	**3.5**	**39**	**0.16**	**127**
DINNER — Beef tenderloin steak, Fries (regular)							
Dinner							
Beef tenderloin steak	5 oz.	25	6	6	13		90
Fries, regular	1	17	7	1	9		12
Total		**42**	**13**	**7**	**22**	**0.54**	**102**
Total Daily Intake		**125**	**44**	**11.5**	**70**	**0.26**	**489**

Low-Saturated-Fat Menu at Home

BREAKFAST	LUNCH	DINNER
English Muffin (1)	Turkey (1 oz.)	Fish (5 oz.)
Canadian Bacon (1 oz.)	Bread (2 slices)	Mashed Potatoes (½ cup)
Milk, skim (8 oz.)	Salad Dressing (1 tsp.)	Corn (½ cup)
Soft Tub Margarine (2 tsp.)	Chips (½ cup)	Tossed Salad (1 cup)
Orange Juice (4 oz.)	Zucchini Cake (1 serving)	Dressing (1 tbsp.)
		Soft Tub Margarine (1 tsp.)
		Sherbet (½ cup)

	Amount	Total Fat (g)	Saturated Fat (g)	Polyunsaturated Fat (g)	Monounsaturated Fat (g)	Saturated Fat Ratio	Cholesterol (mg)
Breakfast							
English muffin	1						
Canadian bacon	1 oz.	3.0	1	0	2		25
Milk, skim	8 oz.	0.5	0	0	0		5
Soft tub margarine	2 tsp.	6.0	1	3	2		
Orange juice	4 oz.		0				
Total		**9.5**	**2**	**3**	**4**	**1.5**	**30**
Lunch							
Turkey	2 oz.	2	1.0	0.5	1.0		44
Bread	2 slices						
Salad dressing	1 tsp.	2	0	1.0	0.5		1
Potato chips	1 cup	10	1.0	6.0	2.0		
Zucchini cake (made w/oil)	1 serving	5	0.5	3.0	1.0		
Total		**19**	**2.5**	**10.5**	**4.5**	**4.2**	**45**

	Amount	Total Fat (g)	Saturated Fat (g)	Polyunsaturated Fat (g)	Monounsaturated Fat (g)	Saturated Fat Ratio	Cholesterol (mg)
Dinner							
Fish (6% fat)	5 oz.	6	1.5	1	3		113
Mashed potatoes	½ cup	4	1.0	2	1		
Corn	½ cup	4	1.0	2	1		
Tossed salad	1 cup						
Dressing	1 tbsp.	5	1.0	2	2		
Soft tub margarine	1 tsp.	3	0.5	1	1		
Sherbet	½ cup						
Total		**22**	**5**	**8**	**8**	**1.6**	**113**
Total Daily Intake		**50.5**	**9.5**	**21.5**	**16.5**	**2.26**	**188**

Chapter 9
Deli and Sub Meals

Sandwiches and subs are a way of life for people on the run. Lots of calories, fat, and sodium can be packed between two slices of bread or into a hoagie bun.

Fixing a sandwich with more lettuce, tomato, and onions can help reduce the fat and sodium content. A heavy hand with the cheese, mayonnaise, and fatty meats adds calories and saturated fats.

Cruising into a Schlotzsky's Deli or a Subway can be faster than making your own sandwich, but take a look at the nutrient content before you choose your sandwich. The comparison of Subway choices can be found in the "Fast-Food Comparison" section. Portion size makes a significant difference in calories, total fat, saturated fats, and sodium.

The Dijon Chicken (10 ounces) sandwich can fit into a healthy meal plan as a quick lunch or late-night supper. Even the Dijon Chicken (15 ounces) can be respectably calculated into a daily nutrition regime. When cheese is the primary protein (The Vegetarian) or added to a high-fat meat sandwich (Corned Beef Reuben), however, the total fat and saturated fat content in one sandwich equals a full day's amount.

Deli meats such as corned beef and bacon can lead to one sandwich containing an entire day's recommended sodium level. Keeping a sandwich choice to under 2,000 milligrams sodium allows for 1,000 to 1,500 milligrams sodium to be consumed at other meals.

Schlotzsky's Deli

	Calories	Total Fat (g)	Saturated Fat (g)	Sodium (mg)
Albacore Tuna (13 oz.)	530	16	4	1,660
Corned Beef Reuben (15 oz.)	830	35	13	3,510
Dijon Chicken (10 oz.)	330	4	1	1,370
Dijon Chicken (15 oz.)	500	6	1	2,090
Roast Beef (14 oz.)	620	17	3	1,730
The Vegetarian (12 oz.)	520	17	7	1,330
Turkey & Bacon Club (17 oz.)	870	40	15	3,010

Subway meals tend to be healthier than Schlotsky's Deli meals. Here is a Subway selection containing 616 calories that fits within the guidelines for total fat, saturated fat, and sodium.

Portion control is made easy at any of over 12,000 Subways throughout the United States. Keep to the 6-inch sub and request low-fat salad dressings, light mayonnaise, and no cheese to keep within healthy guidelines.

Subway

	Calories	Total Fat (g)	Saturated Fat (g)	Sodium (mg)
6-inch Subway Club Sandwich				
1 bag Baked Lays Chips				
Oatmeal Raisin Cookie				
Total	616	15	4	1,600

Supermarket deli sandwiches can also offer ready-to-eat convenience meals. Some of these deli selections feature lower sodium and fat. The comparison on page 152 is an example of the difference in sodium between 2-ounce turkey selections.

Deli Meats Nutrition Facts (2 ounces)

	Calories	Total Fat (g)	Saturated Fat (g)	Cholesterol (mg)	Sodium (mg)
Beef Products					
Bottom round roast	80	3.5	1	30	250
Corned beef bottom round	80	3.0	1	30	450
Pastrami beef bottom round	80	3.0	1	30	480
Peppered beef bottom round	80	3.0	1	30	490
Top round roast	80	2.5	1	30	260
Ham Products					
Cooked ham and water	60	2	1	25	540
Cooked ham and water (lower sodium)	60	2	1	25	330
Luncheon Meats					
Beef bologna	160	13	6.0	30	390
Braunschweiger	170	14	5.0	95	560
Garlic beef bologna	160	13	6.0	30	410
German brand bologna	140	12	4.5	30	420
Liverwurst	170	14	5.0	95	560
Old-fashioned loaf	130	11	4.0	30	380
Olive loaf	120	9	3.5	20	550
Pickle and pimento loaf	130	10	4.0	25	370
Salami	160	13	5.0	35	450
Poultry Products					
Hickory-smoked turkey breast	50	0	0	25	490
Oven-roasted turkey breast	50	0	0	25	420
Oven-roasted turkey breast (lower sodium)	50	0	0	25	270
Smoked tavern chicken breast	70	1	0	35	350

Oven-roasted turkey breast   420 mg. sodium
Oven-roasted turkey breast, low sodium   270 mg. sodium
Hickory-smoked turkey breast   490 mg. sodium

Although ham is higher in sodium than turkey and beef, it is a lower-fat choice than popular luncheon meats. A total fat and saturated fat comparison shows why ham is the nutritional choice.

2-ounce Portion	Total Fat (g)	Saturated Fat (g)
Beef bologna	13	6
Cooked ham & water	2	1
Liverwurst	14	5
Olive loaf	9	3.5
Salami	13	5

Chapter 10
Fast-Food Comparisons

*L*ifestyles today are busier than ever before. Consumers are eating away from home more often and are relying on fast-food restaurants to provide quick and nutritious food choices.

Several national food chain restaurants are included in this analysis of fast foods. Not all items available on the menus are included, but this representative sample should allow for comparative shopping before arriving at the restaurant. Nutrient values have been rounded to whole numbers for easier comparison.

Menus have greatly expanded beyond the hamburgers, cheeseburgers, and fries of the past. Today, many fast-food chain restaurants include vegetarian selections, and poultry items rival the red meat choices. Wendy's restaurants offer salad selections that provide all the food groups for a healthy, personalized meal.

Remember that drive-through ordering can be intimidating if a healthy choice is not made *before* placing the order.

Arby's

Food Item	Serving Size	Calories	Fat (g)	Sodium (mg)	Carbohy- drates (g)
Apple Turnover	1	330	14	180	48
Arby's Melt with Cheese	1	368	18	937	36
Bac'n Cheddar Deluxe	1	539	34	1,140	38
Beef 'n Cheddar	1	507	28	1,216	40
Blue Cheese Dressing	1	290	31	580	2
Blueberry Muffin	1	230	9	290	35
Breaded Chicken Fillet	1	536	28	1,016	46
Broccoli 'n Cheddar Baked Potato	1	571	20	565	89
Cheddar Curly Fries	1 serving	333	18	1,016	40
Chicken Fingers	2 pieces	290	16	677	20
Chocolate Chip Cookie	1	125	6	85	16
Chocolate Shake	1	451	12	341	76
Cinnamon Nut Danish	1	360	11	105	60
Curly Fries	1 serving	300	15	853	38
Deluxe Baked Potato	1	736	36	499	86
Egg Portion	1	95	8	54	6
Fish Fillet	1	529	27	864	50
French Dip	1	475	22	1,411	40
French Toastix	6 pieces	430	21	550	52
Garden Salad	1	61	0.5	40	12
Giant Roast Beef	1	555	28	1,561	43
Grilled Chicken BBQ	1	388	13	1,002	47
Ham 'n Cheese Melt	1	329	13	1,013	34
Home Style Fries	small	212	10	414	29
Home Style Fries	medium	340	156	665	46
Home Style Fries	large	423	19	828	57
Honey French Dressing	1	280	23	400	18
Italian Sub	1	633	36	2,089	46
Junior Roast Beef	1	324	14	779	35
Philly Beef 'n Swiss	1	755	47	2,025	48
Plain Baked Potato	1	355	0	26	82
Plain Croissant	1	220	12	230	25
Reduced-Calorie Buttermilk Ranch Dressing	1	50	15	710	12
Reduced-Calorie Italian Dressing	1	20	1	1,000	3
Regular Roast Beef	1	388	19	1,009	33
Roast Beef Deluxe	1	296	10	826	33
Roast Chicken Club	1	546	31	1,103	37

Food Item	Serving Size	Calories	Fat (g)	Sodium (mg)	Carbohy- drates (g)
Roast Chicken Deluxe on Sesame Seed Bun	1	433	22	763	36
Roast Chicken Salad	1	149	2	418	12
Roast Turkey Deluxe	1	260	7	1,262	33
Super Roast Beef	1	523	27	1,189	50
Table Syrup	1	100	0	30	25
Thousand Island Dressing	1	260	26	420	7
Triple Cheese Melt	1	720	45	1,797	46
Turkey Sub	1	550	27	2,084	47
Vanilla Shake	1	360	12	281	50

Boston Market

Food Item	Serving Size	Calories	Fat (g)	Sodium (mg)	Carbohy- drates (g)
¼ Chicken w/skin	1	630	37	960	2
¼ White Meat Chicken w/Corn Bread, Steamed Vegetables, & Fruit Salad, low-fat, skin & wing removed by customer	1 each	450	10	770	54
¼ White Meat Chicken w/Corn Bread, Steamed Vegetables & Whole Kernel Corn	1 serving	660	16	1,050	89
¼ Dark Meat Chicken w/skin	1	330	22	460	2
¼ Dark Meat Chicken w/o skin	1	210	10	320	1
¼ White Meat Chicken w/skin	1	330	17	530	2
¼ White Meat Chicken w/o skin or wing	1	160	4	350	0
BBQ Baked Beans	¾ cup	330	9	630	53
Brownie	1	450	27	190	47
Butternut Squash, low-fat	¾ cup	160	6	580	25
Caesar Salad Entrée w/Dressing	1 each	520	43	1,420	16
Chicken Breast Sandwich & Fruit Salad, low-fat, no cheese or sauce	1 serving	480	5	910	75
Chicken Caesar Salad w/Dressing	1 each	670	47	1,860	16
Chunky Chicken Salad	1 serving	370	27	800	3
Chocolate Chip Cookie	1	340	17	240	48
Cole Slaw	¾ cup	280	16	520	32
Corn Bread	1 loaf	200	6	390	33

Continued overleaf

Boston Market, *continued*

Food Item	Serving Size	Calories	Fat (g)	Sodium (mg)	Carbohy-drates (g)
Creamed Spinach	¾ cup	280	21	820	12
Fruit Salad, low-fat	¾ cup	70	1	10	17
Garlic and Dill New Potatoes, low-fat	¾ cup	130	3	150	25
Green Bean Casserole	¾ cup	90	5	580	10
Ham & Turkey Club w/Cheese & Sauce	1	890	44	2,350	76
Ham & Turkey Club w/o Cheese & Sauce	1	430	6	1,330	64
Homestyle Mashed Potatoes & Gravy	¾ cup	200	9	560	27
Honey Wheat Roll	1	300	3	560	58
Macaroni and Cheese	¾ cup	280	10	760	36
Mashed Potatoes	⅔ cup	180	8	390	25
Meat Loaf & Brown Gravy	1 serving	390	22	1,040	19
Mediterranean Pasta Salad	¾ cup	170	10	490	16
Original Chicken Pot Pie	1	750	34	2,380	78
Skinless Rotisserie Turkey Breast, low-fat	1	170	1	850	1
Steamed Vegetables, low-fat	⅔ cup	35	1	35	7
Tortellini Salad	¾ cup	380	24	530	29
Turkey Breast Sandwich & Fruit Salad, low-fat, no cheese or sauce	1 serving	460	4	1,070	75
Whole Kernel Corn, low-fat	¾ cup	180	4	170	30

Burger King

Food Item	Serving Size	Calories	Fat (g)	Sodium (mg)	Carbohy-drates (g)
BK Big Fish™	1	700	41	980	56
BK Broiler® Chicken	1	550	29	480	41
Biscuit with Bacon, Egg & Cheese	1	520	31	1,530	39
Biscuit with Sausage	1	590	40	1,390	41
Broiled Chicken Salad	1 serving	200	10	110	7
Cheeseburger	1	380	19	770	28
Chicken Tenders®	8 pieces	310	17	710	19

Food Item	Serving Size	Calories	Fat (g)	Sodium (mg)	Carbohy-drates (g)
Chocolate Shake	1 medium	440	10	333	75
Coated French Fries (salted)	1 medium	340	17	680	43
Croissan'wich® w/Sausage, Egg & Cheese	1	600	46	1,140	25
Double Cheeseburger with Bacon	1	640	39	1,240	28
Double Whopper	1	870	56	940	45
Dutch Apple Pie	1	300	15	230	39
French Dressing	1	140	10	190	11
French Fries (salted)	1 medium	370	20	240	43
French Toast Sticks	1 serving	500	27	490	60
Hamburger	1	330	15	530	28
Hash Browns	1 serving	220	12	320	25
Onion Rings	1 serving	310	14	810	41
Ranch Dressing	1	180	19	170	2
Reduced Calorie Light Italian Dressing	1	15	1	50	3
Thousand Island Dressing	1	140	12	190	7
Vanilla Shake	1 medium	430	9	333	73
Whopper	1	640	39	870	45
Whopper Jr.	1	420	24	530	29

Dairy Queen

Food Item	Serving Size	Calories	Fat (g)	Sodium (mg)	Carbohy-drates (g)
Chicken Breast Fillet Sandwich	1	430	20	760	37
Chili 'n' Cheese Dog	1	330	21	1,090	22
Chocolate Chip Cookie Dough Blizzard®	1 small	660	24	440	99
Chocolate Cone	1 small	240	8	115	37
DQ® Chocolate Soft Serve	1 serving	150	5	75	22
DQ Homestyle® Cheeseburger	1	340	17	850	29
DQ Homestyle® Hamburger	1	290	12	630	29
DQ® (no-fat) Frozen Yogurt	1 serving	100	0	70	21
DQ® Vanilla Orange Bar (no sugar added)	1	60	0	40	17
DQ® Vanilla Soft Serve	1 serving	140	5	70	22
Dipped Cone	1 small	340	17	140	42
Hot Dog	1	240	14	730	19
French Fries	1 small	350	18	630	42

Continued overleaf

Dairy Queen, *continued*

Food Item	Serving Size	Calories	Fat (g)	Sodium (mg)	Carbohy-drates (g)
French Fries	1 large	440	23	790	53
Grilled Chicken Breast Fillet	1	310	10	1,040	30
Heath Breeze®	1 small	470	10	380	85
Onion Rings	1 serving	320	16	180	39
Vanilla Cone	1 small	230	7	115	38
Yogurt Cone	1 medium	260	1	160	56

Domino's

Food Item	Serving Size	Calories	Fat (g)	Sodium (mg)	Carbohy-drates (g)
Anchovies topping only, 6 inches	1 serving	45	2	790	0
Bacon topping only, 12 inches	1 serving	82	7	226	0
Bacon topping only, 14 inches	1 serving	75	6	207	0
Barbeque Buffalo Wings	1 piece	50	1	175	2
Breadsticks	1	78	3	149	11
Cheese only, 6 inches	1	595	28	1,300	68
Cheese only, 12 inches	2 of 8 slices	477	22	1,086	55
Cheese only, 14 inches	2 of 12 slices	455	20	1,029	54
Extra cheese topping only, 6 inches	1 serving	59	5	150	0
Extra cheese topping only, 12 inches	1 serving	48	4	150	1
Extra cheese topping only, 14 inches	1 serving	45	4	140	1
Fresh mushrooms topping only, 12 inches	1 serving	4	0	1	1
Green peppers topping only, 2 inches	1 serving	3	0	0	1
Pepperoni topping only, 12 inches	1 serving	75	7	239	0
Pepperoni topping only, 14 inches	1 serving	66	6	212	0

Hardee's

Food Item	Serving Size	Calories	Fat (g)	Sodium (mg)	Carbohy-drates (g)
Apple Cinnamon 'n Raisin Biscuit	1	200	8	360	30
Bacon & Egg Biscuit	1	570	33	1,400	45
Baked Beans	1 serving	170	1	600	32
Big Cookie™	1	280	12	150	41
Big Roast Beef™	1	460	24	1,230	35
Cheeseburger	1	310	14	890	30
Chicken Breast	1	370	15	1,190	29
Chicken Fillet Sandwich	1	480	18	1,280	54
Chicken Leg	1	170	7	570	15
Chicken Thigh	1	330	15	1,000	30
Chicken Wing	1	200	8	740	23
Chocolate Shake	1	370	5	270	57
Cole Slaw	1 serving	240	20	340	13
Fat-Free French Dressing	1	70	0	580	17
Fisherman's Fillet	1	560	27	1,330	54
French Fries	1 small	240	10	100	33
French Fries	1 medium	350	15	150	49
French Fries	1 large	430	18	190	59
Grilled Chicken Salad	1 serving	150	3	610	11
Grilled Chicken Sandwich	1	350	11	950	38
Ham, Egg & Cheese Biscuit	1	540	30	1,660	48
Hamburger	1	270	11	670	29
Hot Fudge Sundae	1	290	6	310	51
Mashed Potatoes	1 serving	70	0	330	14
Ranch Dressing	1	290	29	510	6
Regular Hash Rounds™	16 pieces	230	14	560	24
Regular Roast Beef	1	320	16	820	26
Sausage Biscuit	1	520	31	1,360	44
Sausage & Egg Biscuit	1	630	40	1,448	45
The Boss™	1	570	33	910	42
Thousand Island Dressing	1	250	23	540	9
Three Pancakes	3	280	2	890	56
Vanilla Shake	1	350	5	300	65

Kentucky Fried Chicken

Food Item	Serving Size	Calories	Fat (g)	Sodium (mg)	Carbohy- drates (g)
BBQ Baked Beans	1 serving	190	3	760	33
Biscuit	1	180	10	560	20
Chunky Chicken Pot Pie	1	770	42	2,160	69
Cole Slaw	1 serving	180	9	280	21
Corn on the Cob	1	150	2	20	35
Cornbread	1	228	13	194	25
Green Beans	1 serving	45	2	730	7
Hot and Spicy Chicken Breast	1	530	35	1,110	23
Hot and Spicy Chicken Drumstick	1	190	11	300	10
Hot and Spicy Chicken Thigh	1	370	27	570	13
Hot and Spicy Chicken Whole Wing	1	210	15	340	9
Hot Wings™ Pieces	6	471	33	1,230	18
Macaroni and Cheese	1 serving	180	8	860	21
Mashed Potatoes with Gravy	1 serving	120	6	440	17
Original Recipe® Breast	1	400	24	1,116	16
Original Recipe® Chicken Sandwich	1	497	22	1,213	46
Original Recipe® Drumstick	1	140	9	422	4
Original Recipe® Thigh	1	250	18	747	6
Original Recipe® Whole Wing	1	140	10	414	5
Potato Salad	1 serving	230	14	540	23
Tender Roast® Breast w/skin	1	251	11	830	2
Tender Roast® Breast w/o skin	1	169	4	797	118
Tender Roast® Drumstick w/skin	1	97	4	271	55
Tender Roast® Drumstick w/o skin	1	67	2	259	0
Tender Roast® Thigh w/skin	1	207	12	504	1
Tender Roast® Thigh w/o skin	1	106	6	312	0
Tender Roast® Wing w/skin	1	121	8	331	1

Long John Silver's

Food Item	Serving Size	Calories	Fat (g)	Sodium (mg)	Carbohy- drates (g)
Batter-Dipped Chicken	1 piece	120	6	400	11
Batter-Dipped Fish	1 piece	170	11	470	12
Batter-Dipped Shrimp	1 piece	35	3	95	2
Breaded Clams	1 serving	300	17	670	31
Cheese Sticks	1 serving	160	9	360	12

Food Item	Serving Size	Calories	Fat (g)	Sodium (mg)	Carbohy-drates (g)
Corn Cobbette w/butter	1	140	8	0	19
Fat-free French Dressing	1	50	0	360	14
Fat-free Ranch Dressing	1	50	0	380	13
Flavorbaked™ Chicken	1 piece	110	3	600	0
Flavorbaked™ Chicken Sandwich	1	290	10	970	27
Flavorbaked™ Fish	1 piece	90	3	320	1
Flavorbaked™ Fish Sandwich	1	320	14	930	28
French Fries	1 small	250	15	500	28
Grab 'n Go Battered Chicken	1	320	12	850	41
Grab 'n Go Battered Chicken w/Cheese	1	370	17	1,090	41
Grab 'n Go Battered Fish	1	300	11	770	39
Grab 'n Go Battered Fish w/Cheese	1	350	16	1,010	39
Hushpuppy	1 piece	60	3	25	9
Italian Dressing	1	130	14	280	2
Popcorn Shrimp Munchers	1 serving	320	15	1,440	33
Ranch Dressing	1	170	18	260	1
Rice	1 serving	140	3	210	26
Side Salad	1	25	0	15	4
Slaw	1 serving	140	6	260	20
Ultimate Fish Sandwich	1	430	21	1,340	44

McDonald's

Food Item	Serving Size	Calories	Fat (g)	Sodium (mg)	Carbohy-drates (g)
Apple Danish	1	360	16	290	51
Bacon, Egg and Cheese Biscuit	1	440	26	1,310	33
Baked Apple Pie	1	260	13	200	34
Big Mac	1	560	31	1,070	45
Breakfast Burrito	1	320	20	600	23
Caesar Dressing	1	160	14	450	7
Cheeseburger	1	320	14	820	35
Chicken McNuggets	4 pieces	190	11	340	10
Chocolate Chip Cookies	1	170	10	120	22
Cinnamon Roll	1	400	20	340	47
Chocolate Shake	1	360	9	250	60
Crispy Chicken Deluxe™	1	500	25	1,100	43
Quarter Pounder	1	420	21	820	37

Continued overleaf

McDonald's, *continued*

Food Item	Serving Size	Calories	Fat (g)	Sodium (mg)	Carbohy-drates (g)
Egg McMuffin®	1	290	12	710	27
Fat-Free Herb Vinaigrette	1	50	0	330	11
Fish Fillet Deluxe™	1	560	28	1,060	54
French Fries	1 small	210	10	135	26
French Fries	1 large	450	22	290	57
Grilled Chicken Deluxe™	1	440	20	1,040	38
Grilled Chicken Salad Deluxe	1 serving	120	2	240	7
Hamburger	1	270	10	580	34
Hash Browns	1	130	8	330	14
Hot Fudge Sundae	1	340	12	170	52
Hotcakes (Plain)	1 serving	310	7	610	53
Ranch Dressing	1	230	21	500	10
Red French Reduced-Calorie Dressing	1	160	8	490	23
Sausage Biscuit w/Egg	1	510	35	1,210	33
Sausage McMuffin®	1	360	23	470	26
Scrambled Eggs	1 serving	160	11	170	1
Vanilla Reduced-Fat Ice Cream Cone	1	150	5	75	23
Vanilla Shake	1	360	9	250	59

Pizza Hut

Food Item	Serving Size	Calories	Fat (g)	Sodium (mg)	Carbohy-drates (g)
Apple Dessert Pizza	1 slice	250	5	230	48
Beef Topping Pan Pizza	1 slice	310	14	720	31
Bread Stick	1	130	4	170	20
Cheese Pan Pizza	1 slice	300	14	610	30
Chicken Supreme Pan Pizza	1 slice	280	11	570	32
Chicken Supreme Pizza	1 slice	220	7	550	26
Garlic Bread	1 slice	140	8	240	16
Ham Pan Pizza	1 slice	250	9	590	31
Italian Sausage Pan Pizza	1 slice	350	18	740	31
Meat Lover's® Pan Pizza	1 slice	360	19	870	30
Mild Buffalo Wings	5 pieces	200	12	510	<1
Pepperoni Lover's® Pan Pizza	1 slice	350	17	800	32
Pepperoni Pan Pizza	1 slice	280	12	640	31
Pork Topping Pan Pizza	1 slice	300	13	720	31
Thin 'N Crispy® Beef Topping Pizza	1 slice	240	11	790	22
Thin 'N Crispy® Cheese Pizza	1 slice	210	9	530	21

Food Item	Serving Size	Calories	Fat (g)	Sodium (mg)	Carbohy- drates (g)
Thin 'N Crispy® Ham Pizza	1 slice	190	6	560	23
Thin 'N Crispy® Italian Sausage Pizza	1 slice	300	16	740	24
Thin 'N Crispy® Meat Lover's® Pizza	1 slice	310	16	900	25
Thin 'N Crispy® Pepperoni Pizza	1 slice	220	9	610	22
Thin 'N Crispy® Pepperoni Lover's® Pizza	1 slice	270	12	780	26
Thin 'N Crispy® Pork Topping Pizza	1 slice	270	13	780	22
Thin 'N Crispy® Super Supreme Pizza	1 slice	280	13	810	26
Thin 'N Crispy® Supreme Pizza	1 slice	250	11	710	24
Thin 'N Crispy® Veggie Lover's® Pizza	1 slice	170	6	460	23
Super Supreme Pan Pizza	1 slice	340	16	790	33
Supreme Pan Pizza	1 slice	300	13	670	32
Spaghetti with Marinara	1 serving	490	6	730	91
Spaghetti w/Meat Sauce	1 serving	600	13	910	98
Spaghetti w/Meatballs	1 serving	850	24	1,120	120
Veggie Lover's® Pan Pizza	1 slice	240	9	480	31

Subway

Food Item	Serving Size	Calories	Fat (g)	Sodium (mg)	Carbohy- drates (g)
B.L.T. on wheat	6 inches	327	10	957	44
Chicken Taco Sub on white w/o cheese or condiments	6 inches	421	16	1,264	43
Cold Cut Trio on white	6 inches	362	13	1,401	39
Ham on wheat	6 inches	302	5	1,308	45
Ham Sandwich	1	234	4	773	37
Roast Beef on white	6 inches	288	5	928	39
Roast Beef Sandwich	1	245	4	638	38
Roasted Chicken Breast on wheat	6 inches	348	6	978	47
Spicy Italian on wheat	6 inches	482	25	1,604	44
Steak & Cheese on wheat w/o cheese or condiments	6 inches	398	10	1,117	47
Subway Club® on white	6 inches	297	5	1,341	40

Continued overleaf

Subway, *continued*

Food Item	Serving Size	Calories	Fat (g)	Sodium (mg)	Carbohy-drates (g)
Subway Seafood & Crab® on white	6 inches	415	19	849	38
Subway Seafood & Crab® w/light mayonnaise dressing on wheat	6 inches	347	10	884	45
Tuna on white	6 inches	527	32	875	38
Tuna w/light mayonnaise dressing on white	6 inches	376	15	928	39
Turkey Breast and Ham on white	6 inches	280	4	1,350	39
Turkey Breast on white	6 inches	273	4	1,391	40
Turkey Breast Sandwich	1	235	4	944	38
Veggie Delight™ on wheat	6 inches	237	3	593	44

Taco Bell

Food Item	Serving Size	Calories	Fat (g)	Sodium (mg)	Carbohy-drates (g)
Bean Burrito	1	380	12	1,100	55
Big Chicken Burrito Supreme®	1	510	24	1,900	52
Burrito Supreme®	1	520	23	1,520	54
Chicken Quesadilla	1	410	22	1,170	34
Choco Taco® Ice Cream Dessert	1	310	17	100	37
Cinnamon Twists	1 serving	140	6	190	19
Double Decker® Taco	1	340	15	750	38
Grilled Chicken Burrito	1	410	15	1,380	50
Grilled Chicken Soft Taco	1	240	12	1,110	21
Grilled Steak Soft Taco	1	230	10	1,020	20
Mexican Pizza	1	570	35	1,040	42
Mexican Rice	1 serving	190	9	760	23
Nachos	1 serving	320	18	570	34
Nachos BellGrande®	1 serving	770	39	1,310	84
Steak Fajita Wrap™	1	470	21	1,190	50
Steak Fajita Wrap™ Supreme®	1	510	25	1,200	52
Taco	1	180	10	330	12
Taco Salad w/salsa	1	850	52	1,780	65
Taco Salad w/salsa w/o shell	1	420	22	1,520	32
Taco Supreme™	1	220	14	350	14
Veggie Fajita Wrap™	1	420	19	980	53
Veggie Fajita Wrap™ Supreme®	1	470	22	990	55

Wendy's

Food Item	Serving Size	Calories	Fat (g)	Sodium (mg)	Carbohy-drates (g)
Bacon & Cheese Baked Potato	1	530	18	1,390	78
Big Bacon Classic	1	580	30	1,460	46
Breaded Chicken Sandwich	1	440	18	840	44
Broccoli & Cheese Baked Potato	1	470	14	470	80
Chicken Club Sandwich	1	470	20	970	44
Chili & Cheese Baked Potato	1	630	24	770	83
Chicken Caesar Pita w/dressing	1	490	18	1,320	48
Chicken Nuggets	5 pieces	230	16	470	11
Chicken Salad	2 tbsp.	70	5	135	2
Chocolate Chip Cookie	1	270	13	120	36
Classic Greek Pita w/dressing	1	440	20	1,050	50
Cottage Cheese	2 tbsp.	30	2	125	1
Cucumbers	2 slices	0	0	0	0
Fat-Free French Dressing	2 tbsp.	35	0	150	8
French Fries	1 small	270	13	85	35
French Fries	1 large	470	23	150	61
Frosty™ Dairy Dessert	1 small	330	8	200	56
Garden Ranch Chicken Pita w/dressing	1	480	18	1,180	51
Garden Veggie Pita w/dressing	1	400	17	760	52
Green Peas	2 tbsp.	15	0	25	3
Green Peppers	2 pieces	0	0	0	1
Grilled Chicken Caesar Salad w/o dressing	1	260	9	1,170	17
Grilled Chicken Fillet	1	110	3	450	0
Grilled Chicken Salad w/o dressing	1	200	8	720	9
Grilled Chicken Sandwich	1	310	8	790	35
Hamburger Patty	1	200	14	290	0
Hamburger, Kids' Meal	1	270	10	610	33
Hamburger, plain single	1	360	16	580	31
Iceberg/Romaine Lettuce	1 cup	10	0	5	2
Italian Caesar Dressing	2 tbsp.	150	16	240	1
Italian, Reduced-Fat Reduced-Calorie	2 tbsp.	40	3	340	2
Mushrooms	¼ cup	0	0	0	1
Pasta Salad	2 tbsp.	35	2	180	4
Plain Baked Potato	1	310	0	26	71
Potato Salad	2 tbsp.	80	7	180	5

Continued overleaf

Wendy's, *continued*

Food Item	Serving Size	Calories	Fat (g)	Sodium (mg)	Carbohy- drates (g)
Red Onions	3 rings	0	0	0	1
Sliced Orange	2 slices	15	0	0	4
Sliced Peaches	1 piece	15	0	0	4
Sliced Pepperoni	6 slices	30	3	70	0
Soft Breadstick	1	130	3	250	23
Spicy Chicken Fillet	1	210	9	920	10
Sunflower Seeds & Raisins	2 tbsp.	80	5	0	5
Taco Chips	15	210	11	180	24
Taco Salad w/o dressing	1	380	19	1,040	28
Tomato Wedge	1 piece	5	0	0	1

Appendix

Food Label Terms

Many people do not take the time to read a prepared food label closely to decide if they will like the sauce or ingredients. A brief description of the terms frequently encountered on prepared-food labels can help people decide if the meal will fit their taste.

Adobo sauce A spicy Mexican sauce made from chili peppers, herbs, and vinegar.

A la king A dish of chopped meat (i.e., chicken or turkey) in a cream sauce with mushrooms, pimento, and green peppers.

Alfredo A thick pasta sauce made with Parmesan cheese and cream.

Au gratin: A food or dish topped with grated cheese and/or bread-crumbs.

Cacciatore A term used to describe food prepared with mushrooms, onions, and tomatoes.

Carbonara An Italian term for pasta with a cream sauce containing Parmesan cheese and bacon bits.

Curry An East Indian flavoring that can be used in varying degrees of spiciness.

Fricassee A creamy dish of meat (i.e., chicken or turkey) and vegetables in a white cream sauce.

Marengo An Italian term used to describe chicken or veal that has been sautéed in oil and braised with onions, tomatoes, olives, and garlic.

Marinara A tomato sauce with garlic, oregano, and sometimes onions.

Parmigiana A term used to describe food cooked with Parmesan cheese.

Pesto An uncooked sauce made from fresh basil, garlic, pine nuts, Parmesan cheese, and olive oil.

Piccata An Italian term used to describe chicken or veal that is sliced thinly, sautéed, and served in a sauce made from lemon juice and chopped parsley.

Primavera An Italian term describing dishes made with a variety of vegetables.

Scaloppine An Italian term used to describe a thin slice of meat that has been coated with flour and sautéed. These dishes are served with a sauce made from white wine and tomatoes.

Teriyaki A Japanese dish of beef, chicken, or vegetables that have been marinated in a mixture of soy sauce, sugar, saké, ginger, and other seasonings before grilling or broiling.

Vinaigrette A sauce made from oil and vinegar.

Exchange List for Meal Planning

Exchange lists have been produced by the American Diabetes Association and the American Dietetic Association to aid in meal planning. Foods are grouped together based on their similarities in carbohydrate, protein, and fat content. Serving sizes for a stated food are indicated.

Some of the foods listed here are provided for reference in assessing how prepared foods can be used in your diabetes meal plan.

Starch List

Each food in this list contains about 15 grams of carbohydrate, 3 grams of protein, 1 gram or less of fat, and about 80 calories per serving. In general, one starch exchange is

- ½ cup cereal, pasta, or starchy vegetable
- 1 ounce of a bread product or one slice of bread
- ¾ to 1 ounce of most snack foods (some snack foods may have extra fat)

Breads

Food Item	Serving Size
Bagel	½ (1 ounce)
Bread, reduced calorie	2 slices (1½ ounces)
Bread, white, whole wheat, pumpernickel, rye	1 slice (1 ounce)
Bread sticks, crisp, 4 in. long × ½ in.	2 (⅔ ounce)
English muffin	½
Hog dog or hamburger bun	½ (1 ounce)
Pita, 6 in. across	½
Raisin bread, unfrosted	1 slice (1 ounce)
Roll, plain, small	1 (1 ounce)
Tortilla, corn, 6 in. across	1
Tortilla, flour, 7–8 in. across	1
Waffle, 4½ in. square, reduced-fat	1

Cereals and Grains

Food Item	Serving Size
Bran cereals	½ cup
Bulgur	½ cup
Cereals, cooked	½ cup
Cereals, unsweetened, ready to eat	¾ cup
Cornmeal (dry)	3 tablespoons
Couscous	⅓ cup
Flour (dry)	3 tablespoons
Granola, low fat	¼ cup

Continued overleaf

Cereals and Grains, *continued*

Food Item	Serving Size
Grape-Nuts	¼ cup
Grits	½ cup
Kasha	½ cup
Millet	¼ cup
Muesli	¼ cup
Oats	½ cup
Pasta	½ cup
Puffed cereal	1½ cups
Rice, white or brown	⅓ cup
Rice milk	½ cup
Shredded Wheat	½ cup
Sugar-frosted cereal	½ cup
Wheat germ	3 tablespoons

Starchy Vegetables

Food Item	Serving Size
Baked beans	⅓ cup
Corn	½ cup
Corn on cob, medium	1 (5 ounces)
Mixed vegetables with corn, peas, or pasta	1 cup
Peas, green	½ cup
Plantain	½ cup
Potato, baked or boiled	1 small (3 ounces)
Potato, mashed	½ cup
Squash, winter (acorn, butternut)	1 cup
Yam, sweet potato, plain	½ cup

Crackers and Snacks

Food Item	Serving Size
Animal crackers	8
Graham crackers, 2½ in. square	3
Matzoh	¾ ounce
Melba toast	4 slices
Oyster crackers	24
Popcorn (popped, no fat added or low-fat microwave)	3 cups
Pretzels	¾ ounce

Food Item	Serving Size
Rice cakes, 4 in. across	2
Saltine-type crackers	6
Snack chips, fat free (tortilla, potato)	15–20 (¾ ounce)
Whole wheat crackers, no fat added	2–5 (¾ ounce)

Starchy Foods Prepared with Fat
(Count as 1 Starch Exchange plus 1 Fat Exchange)

Food Item	Serving Size
Biscuit, 2½ in. across	1
Chow mein noodles	½ cup
Cornbread, 2 in. cube	1 (2 ounces)
Crackers, round butter-type	6
Croutons	1 cup
French fried potatoes	16–25 (3 ounces)
Granola	¼ cup
Muffin, small	1 (1½ ounces)
Pancake, 4 in. across	2
Popcorn, microwave (fat added)	3 cups
Sandwich crackers, cheese or peanut butter filling	3
Stuffing, bread (prepared)	⅓ cup
Taco shell, 6 in. across	2
Waffle, 4½ in. square	1
Whole wheat crackers, fat added	4–6 (1 ounce)

Fruit List

Each food in this list contains about 15 grams of carbohydrate and 60 calories per serving. In general, one fruit exchange is

- One small to medium fresh fruit
- ½ cup canned or fresh fruit or fruit juice
- ¼ cup dried fruit

Fruit

Food Item	Serving Size
Apple, unpeeled, small	1 (4 ounces)
Apples, dried	4 rings
Applesauce, unsweetened	½ cup
Apricots, canned	½ cup
Apricots, dried	8 halves
Apricots, fresh	4 whole (5½ ounces)
Banana, small	1 (4 ounces)
Blackberries	¾ cup
Blueberries	¾ cup
Cantaloupe, small	⅓ melon (11 ounces) *or* 1 cup cubes
Cherries, sweet, canned	½ cup
Cherries, sweet, fresh	12 (3 ounces)
Dates	3
Figs, dried	1½
Figs, fresh	1½ large or 2 medium (3½ ounces)
Fruit cocktail	½ cup
Grapefruit sections, canned	¾ cup
Grapefruit, large	½ (11 ounces)
Grapes, small	17 (3 ounces)
Honeydew melon	1 slice (10 ounces) or 1 cup cubes
Kiwi	1 (3½ ounces)
Mandarin oranges, canned	¾ cup
Mango, small	½ fruit (5½ ounces) or ½ cup
Nectarine, small	1 (5 ounces)
Orange, small	1 (6½ ounces)
Papaya	½ fruit (8 ounces) or 1 cup cubes
Peach, medium, fresh	1 (6 ounces)
Peaches, canned	½ cup
Pear, large, fresh	½ (4 ounces)
Pears, canned	½ cup
Pineapple, canned	½ cup
Pineapple, fresh	¾ cup
Plums, canned	½ cup
Plums, small	2 (5 ounces)
Prunes, dried	3
Raisins	2 tablespoons

Food Item	Serving Size
Raspberries	1 cup
Strawberries	1¼ cups whole berries
Tangerines, small	2 (8 ounces)
Watermelon	1 slice (13½ ounces) or 1¼ cups cubes

Fruit Juice

Food Item	Serving Size
Apple juice/cider	½ cup
Cranberry juice cocktail	⅓ cup
Cranberry juice cocktail, reduced-calorie	1 cup
Fruit juice blends, 100% juice	⅓ cup
Grape juice	⅓ cup
Grapefruit juice	½ cup
Orange juice	½ cup
Pineapple juice	½ cup
Prune juice	⅓ cup

Milk List

Each serving of milk or milk product in this list contains about 12 grams of carbohydrate and 8 grams of protein. The amount of fat in the milk (0 to 8 grams per serving) determines whether it is identified as skim/very-low-fat-milk, low-fat milk, or whole milk. In general, one milk is 1 cup.

Skim and Very-Low-Fat Milk
(0–3 grams fat per serving)

Food Item	Serving Size
½% milk	1 cup
1% milk	1 cup
Evaporated skim milk	½ cup
Nonfat dry milk	⅓ cup (dry)

Continued overleaf

Skim and Very-Low-Fat Milk, *continued*
(0–3 grams fat per serving)

Food Item	Serving Size
Nonfat or low-fat buttermilk	1 cup
Nonfat or low-fat fruit-flavored yogurt sweetened w/ aspartame or with a nonnutritive sweetener	1 cup
Plain nonfat yogurt	¾ cup
Skim milk	1 cup

Low-Fat Milk
(5 grams fat per serving)

Food Item	Serving Size
2% milk	1 cup
Plain low-fat yogurt	¾ cup
Sweet acidophilus milk	1 cup

Whole Milk
(8 grams fat per serving)

Food Item	Serving Size
Evaporated whole milk	½ cup
Goat's milk	1 cup
Kefir	1 cup
Whole milk	1 cup

Other Carbohydrates

This group of foods allows for substitution of any food choice on the list for a starch, a fruit, or a milk in the meal plan. These foods can be substituted even though they contain added sugars or fat. Because many of these foods are concentrated sources of carbohydrate and fat, the portion sizes are usually small.

Food	Serving Size	Exchanges Per Serving
Angel food cake, unfrosted	1/12 cake	2 carbohydrates
Brownie, small, unfrosted	2 in. square	1 carbohydrate, 1 fat
Cake, frosted	2 in. square	2 carbohydrates, 1 fat
Cake, unfrosted	2 in. square	1 carbohydrate, 1 fat
Cookie, fat-free	2 small	1 carbohydrate
Cookie or sandwich cookie w/ creme filling	2 small	1 carbohydrate, 1 fat
Cupcake, frosted	1 small	2 carbohydrates, 1 fat
Cranberry sauce, jellied	¼ cup	2 carbohydrates
Doughnut, plain cake	1 medium (1½ ounces)	2 carbohydrates, 2 fats
Doughnut, glazed	3¾ in. across (2 ounces)	2 carbohydrates, 2 fats
Fruit juice bars, frozen, 100% juice	1 bar (3 ounces)	1 carbohydrate
Fruit snacks, chewy (pureed fruit concentrate)	1 roll (¾ ounce)	1 carbohydrate
Fruit spreads, 100% fruit	1 tablespoon	1 carbohydrate
Gelatin, regular	½ cup	1 carbohydrate
Gingersnaps	3	1 carbohydrate
Granola bar	1 bar	1 carbohydrate, 1 fat
Granola bar, fat-free	1 bar	2 carbohydrates
Hummus	⅓ cup	1 carbohydrate, 1 fat
Ice cream	½ cup	1 carbohydrate, 2 fats
Ice cream, fat-free, no sugar added	½ cup	1 carbohydrate
Ice cream, light	½ cup	1 carbohydrate, 1 fat
Jam or jelly, regular	1 tablespoon	1 carbohydrate
Milk, chocolate, whole	1 cup	2 carbohydrates, 1 fat
Pie, fruit, 2 crusts	⅙ pie	3 carbohydrates, 2 fats
Pie, pumpkin or custard	⅛ pie	1 carbohydrate, 2 fats
Potato chips	12–18 (1 ounce)	1 carbohydrate, 2 fats
Pudding, regular (made with low-fat milk)	½ cup	2 carbohydrates
Pudding, sugar-free (made with low-fat milk)	½ cup	1 carbohydrate
Salad dressing, fat-free	¼ cup	1 carbohydrate
Sherbet, sorbet	½ cup	2 carbohydrates
Spaghetti or pasta sauce, canned	½ cup	1 carbohydrate, 1 fat
Sweet roll or Danish	1 (2½ ounces)	2½ carbohydrates, 2 fats
Syrup, light	2 tablespoons	1 carbohydrate
Syrup, regular	1 tablespoon	1 carbohydrate
Syrup, regular	¼ cup	4 carbohydrates
Tortilla chips	6–12 (1 ounce)	1 carbohydrate, 2 fats

Continued overleaf

Other Carbohyydrates, *continued*

Food Item		Serving Size
Yogurt, frozen, fat-free, no sugar added	½ cup	1 carbohydrate
Yogurt, frozen, low-fat, fat-free	⅓ cup	1 carbohydrate, 0–1 fat
Yogurt, low-fat with fruit	1 cup	3 carbohydrates, 0–1 fat
Vanilla wafers	5	1 carbohydrate, 1 fat

Meat and Meat Substitutes List

Very Lean Meat and Substitutes List

Food Item	Serving Size
Poultry: Chicken or turkey (white meat, no skin), Cornish hen (no skin)	1 ounce
Fish: Fresh or frozen cod, flounder, haddock, halibut, trout; tuna fresh or canned in water	1 ounce
Shellfish: Clams, crab, lobster, scallops, shrimp, imitation shellfish	1 ounce
Game: Duck or pheasant (no skin), venison, buffalo, ostrich	1 ounce
Cheese: 1 gram or less fat per ounce	
Nonfat or low-fat cottage cheese	¼ cup
Fat-free cheese	1 ounce
Other:	
Processed sandwich meats w/1 gram or less fat per ounce, such as deli thin, shaved meats, chipped beef, or turkey ham	1 ounce
Egg whites	2
Egg substitutes, plain	¼ cup
Hot dogs w/1 gram or less fat per ounce	1 ounce
Kidney (high in cholesterol)	1 ounce
Sausage w/1 gram or less fat per ounce	1 ounce

Lean Meat and Substitutes List

Food Item	Serving Size
Beef: USDA Select or Choice grades of lean beef trimmed of fat, such as round, sirloin, and flank steak; tenderloin; roast (rib, chuck, rump); steak (T-bone, porterhouse, cubed), or ground round	1 ounce

Food Item	Serving Size
Pork: Lean pork, such as fresh ham; canned, cured, or boiled ham; Canadian bacon; or tenderloin or center loin chop	1 ounce
Lamb: Roast, chop, leg	1 ounce
Veal: Lean chop, roast	1 ounce
Poultry: Chicken, turkey (dark meat, no skin), chicken white meat (w/skin), domestic duck or goose (well drained of fat, no skin)	1 ounce
Fish	
Herring (uncreamed or smoked)	1 ounce
Oysters	6 medium
Salmon (fresh or canned), catfish	1 ounce
Sardines (canned)	2 medium
Tuna (canned in oil, drained)	1 ounce
Game: Goose (no skin), rabbit	1 ounce
Cheese:	
4.5% fat cottage cheese	¼ cup
Grated Parmesan	2 tablespoons
Cheeses w/3 grams or less fat per ounce	1 ounce
Other:	
Hot dogs with 3 grams or less fat per ounce	1½ ounces
Processed sandwich meat with 3 grams or less fat per ounce, such as turkey pastrami or kielbasa	1 ounce
Liver, heart (high in cholesterol)	1 ounce

Medium-Fat Meat and Substitutes List

Food Item	Serving Size
Beef: Most beef products fall into this category (ground beef, meatloaf, corned beef, short ribs, USDA Prime grades of meat trimmed of fat, such as prime rib)	1 ounce
Pork: Top loin, chop, Boston butt, cutlet	1 ounce
Lamb: Rib roast, ground	1 ounce
Veal: Cutlet (ground or cubed, unbreaded)	1 ounce
Poultry: Chicken dark meat (w/skin), ground turkey or ground chicken, fried chicken (w/skin)	1 ounce
Fish: Any fried fish product	1 ounce
Cheese: With 5 grams or less fat per ounce	
Feta	1 ounce

Continued overleaf

Medium-Fat Meat and Substitutes List, *continued*

Food Item	Serving Size
Mozzarella	1 ounce
Ricotta	¼ cup (2 ounces)
Other:	
Egg (high in cholesterol, limit to three per week)	1
Sausage w/5 grams or less fat per ounce	1 ounce
Soy milk	1 cup
Tempeh	¼ cup
Tofu	4 ounces or ½ cup

High-Fat Meat and Substitutes

Food Item	Serving Size
Pork: Spareribs, ground pork, pork sausage	1 ounce
Cheese: All regular cheeses, such as American, cheddar, Monterey Jack, or Swiss	1 ounce
Other: Processed sandwich meats with 8 grams or less fat per ounce, such as bologna, pimento loaf, or salami	1 ounce
Sausage such as bratwurst, Italian, knockwurst, Polish, or smoked	1 ounce
Hot dog (turkey or chicken)	1 (10 per lb)
Bacon	3 slices (20 slices/lb)

Fat List

Monounsaturated Fats

Food Item	Serving Size
Avocado, medium	⅛ (1 ounce)
Oil (canola, olive, peanut)	1 teaspoon
Olives:	
Green, stuffed	10 large
Ripe (black)	8 large
Nuts:	
Almonds, cashews	6 nuts
Mixed (50% peanuts)	6 nuts
Peanuts	10 nuts
Pecans	4 halves
Peanut butter, smooth or crunchy	2 teaspoons
Sesame seeds	1 tablespoon
Tahini paste	2 teaspoons

Polyunsaturated Fats

Food Item	Serving Size
Margarine:	
Stick, tub, or squeeze	1 teaspoon
Lower fat (30% to 50% vegetable oil)	1 tablespoon
Mayonnaise:	
Regular	1 teaspoon
Reduced-fat	1 tablespoon
Miracle Whip Salad Dressing®:	
Regular	2 teaspoons
Reduced-fat	1 tablespoon
Nuts, walnuts, English	4 halves
Oil (corn, safflower, soybean)	1 teaspoon
Salad dressing:	
Regular	1 tablespoon
Reduced-fat	2 tablespoons
Seeds, pumpkin or sunflower	1 tablespoon

Saturated Fats

Food Item	Serving Size
Bacon, cooked	1 slice
	(20 slices/lb)
Bacon, grease	1 teaspoon
Butter:	
Reduced-fat	1 tablespoon
Stick	1 teaspoon
Whipped	2 teaspoons
Chitterlings, boiled	2 tablespoons
	(½ ounce)
Coconut, sweetened, shredded	2 tablespoons
Cream, half and half	2 tablespoons
Cream cheese:	
Reduced-fat	2 tablespoons
	(1 ounce)
Regular	1 tablespoon
	(½ ounce)
Shortening or lard	1 teaspoon
Sour cream:	
Reduced-fat	3 tablespoons
Regular	2 tablespoons

Glossary

---

*T*his glossary explains terms frequently encountered by people with diabetes. Some of the terms refer to herbal compounds that may be considered in a treatment regime. Others are nutrition terms—such as *calories* and *carbohydrates*—that may need a scientific definition. Terms such as *cholesterol, coronary heart disease*, and *hypertension* are included because these conditions are usually mentioned in the same breath with diabetes.

This glossary can be a handy reference for the diabetes educator and person with diabetes, giving both individuals a common vocabulary while working together as a medical team.

Aloe vera A plant with a sap that has been shown effective in helping lower blood glucose levels. Topical application of this sap has helped heal foot wounds in people with diabetes.

Beta cells Cells in the pancreas that make insulin. These cells are found in the islets of Langerhans.

Bierbock root: A root that contains inulin that helps lower blood glucose levels.

Bitter melon A plant with biological properties to help lower blood glucose and cholesterol levels.

Calories The amount of energy provided by a food is represented in unit terms as a calorie. Energy from foods is derived from digestion of carbohydrates, protein, fats, and alcohol.

Capsaicin (cayenne pepper) A vegetable product that has been shown to help decrease neuropathy pain, especially in peripheral tissues, when applied topically.

Carbohydrates A major source of calories in food that comes from sugar (simple carbohydrates) and starch (complex carbohydrates). Carbohydrates are converted into glucose during digestion and are the major component in foods that affect blood glucose levels. Since 1994, the American Diabetes Association has liberalized its recommendations concerning the use of table sugar in the diabetic diet. Studies showed that blood glucose levels are affected by a number of factors, not just whether a food contained simple or complex carbohydrates. Table sugar ingested as a snack or as part of a meal is not the sole cause of high blood glucose levels.

Cholesterol A fatty substance produced by the liver and used in the human body to build cell walls and make hormones. Eating high levels of saturated fats in the diet is believed to elevate blood cholesterol levels.

Coriander An herb that has been studied in animals for its effects on lowering blood glucose levels.

Coronary heart disease A condition that occurs when the arteries that nourish the heart muscle become narrowed and/or blocked. The heart cannot efficiently pump blood throughout the body when this disease is present.

Dandelion root A vegetable product that contains inulin that may help lower blood glucose levels.

Diabetes mellitus A disease in which the body cannot produce enough insulin or use insulin efficiently enough to maintain a normal blood glucose level.

Fats A source of calories in food coming from animal and plant products. Fats contain twice as many calories per unit as carbohydrates and protein; quantities are frequently limited in meal planning to encourage weight control. Saturated fats are predominately found in animal products; unsaturated fats are mainly from vegetable and seafood sources.

Fenugreek seeds An herb that has been shown in numerous medical studies to reduce blood glucose levels. Many diabetes experts believe that the lowering of blood glucose levels from fenugreek is a result of the fiber in the seeds.

Fiber A component of plants that the human digestive system does not break down. Fruits, vegetables, and legumes (beans, peas) are the main sources of fiber in the diet.

Food exchanges Food groups used in the American Diabetes Association and the American Dietetic Association Exchange Lists for Meal Planning. Foods are divided into seven groups: starches, other carbohydrates, meat and meat substitutes, vegetables, fruit, milk, and fats. Foods in a given group can be exchanged for any other food in the same group for blood glucose management.

Glucose A simple form of sugar produced during the digestion of carbohydrates. The amount of glucose in the blood is referred to as the blood glucose level.

Glycohemoglobin A test that indicates blood glucose levels in the blood during the past 2 to 3 months. The test is frequently referred to as the hemoglobin A1C.

Gymnena An herb used primarily in India for blood glucose control. Gymnena has been shown to have similar activity in the body as tolbutamide (a sulfonylurea used in type 2 diabetes).

Hyperglycemia A condition of high blood glucose (above 250 mg/dl) usually occurring with frequent urination, thirst, and fatigue.

Hypertension or high blood pressure Blood pressure greater than 140/90 mm Hg. The systolic pressure (140) is the highest pressure at the moment the heart contracts and pumps blood into arteries. The diastolic pressure (90) is the lowest pressure in arteries just before the next heart contraction. Current estimates indicate that as many as 25 percent of the adult U.S. population may have hypertension, many with no symptoms. Untreated hypertension can harm body organs, especially the kidneys, when an adequate supply of blood is not supplied to the tissues.

Hypoglycemia Low blood glucose (below 70 mg/dl), frequently called an *insulin reaction*. Symptoms of hypoglycemia are moodiness, mental confusion, shakiness, and dizziness.

Insulin A hormone produced by the pancreas that helps the cells use glucose for energy.

Insulin resistance A condition frequently seen in people with type 2 diabetes in which the body does not properly use insulin.

Nephropathy A condition resulting from diabetes complications that causes the kidneys to not function properly.

Neuropathy A condition resulting from diabetes complications affecting the nerves. Peripheral neuropathy refers to those nerves controlling sensation in the feet, hands, and joints. Autonomic neuropathy relates to nerve function of major organs, such as the digestive tract or urinary tract.

Obesity A condition of abnormal and excessive body fat. Obesity is a major risk factor for the development of type 2 diabetes.

Oral hypoglycemic agents Medications taken by mouth that help lower blood glucose levels. These medications are used by people with type 2 diabetes and are not a form of insulin.

Pancreas An organ of the body that secretes digestive enzymes and hormones (i.e., insulin). A healthy pancreas releases digestive enzymes and insulin when needed to provide nutrients to cells in the body.

Protein A source of calories in the diet that also provides amino acids for cell rebuilding, cell growth, and hormone production. Protein is primarily found in meats, poultry, seafood, eggs, milk, vegetables, and legumes.

Retinopathy A condition resulting in damage to small blood vessels of the eye. Vision impairment results when blood and fluids leak into the retina of the eye.

Sugar or table sugar A form of carbohydrate that provides calories and raises blood glucose levels. Sugar can be identified on food labels as brown sugar, confectioner's sugar, invert sugar, raw sugar, fructose, lactose, sucrose, maltose, dextrose, glucose, honey, corn syrup, molasses, or sorghum.

Sugar alcohols A sweetener used in some "sugar-free" products. These products, called sorbitol, maltitol, and mannitol, contain calories like sugar does.

Sugar substitutes A sweetener used in place of sugar in beverages and recipes. Many sugar substitutes (i.e., saccharin, aspartame, acesulfama-K) have fewer calories than sugar and do not affect blood glucose levels.

Triglycerides Fats found in the body from food eaten or produced by the liver from extra calorie sources such as carbohydrates or alcohol. Elevated triglyceride levels are associated with an increased risk of heart disease.

Type 1 diabetes A form of diabetes that usually develops before age 30. It is caused by an immune system attack on the beta cells in the pancreas. People with type 1 diabetes need to take insulin from another source to survive.

Type 2 diabetes A form of diabetes usually occurring after age 30. Some people cannot produce enough insulin to keep up with their body's needs. Others are insulin resistant and cannot adequately utilize the insulin provided by their pancreas. Diet, exercise, oral medication, and/or insulin may be prescribed to help maintain normal blood glucose levels.

References

ALBRINK, M. J., ET AL. 1986. The beneficial effect of fish oil supplements on serum lipids and clotting function of patients with type 2 diabetes mellitus. *Diabetes* 35 (Supp.): 43A.

ANDERSON, R. A., ET AL. 1983. Chromium supplementation of human subjects: Effects on glucose, insulin, and lipid variables. *Metabolism* 32: 894–99.

———. 1991. Supplemental chromium effects on glucose, insulin, glucagons, and urinary chromium loss in subjects consuming controlled low chromium diets. *American Journal of Clinical Nutrition* 54: 909–16.

BEN, G., ET AL. 1991. Effects of chronic alcohol intake on carbohydrate and lipid metabolism in subjects with type II (non-insulin dependent) diabetes. *American Journal of Medicine* 90: 70.

BERGAMINI, E., ET AL. 1994. Beneficial effects of vanadyl sulfate administration on sugar metabolism in the senescent rat. *Annals of the New York Academy of Science* 717: 174–79.

CAPSAICIN STUDY GROUP. 1992. Effect of treatments with capsaicin on daily activities of patients with painful diabetic neuropathy. *Diabetes Care* 15(2): 159–65.

COLAQIURI, S., ET AL. 1989. Metabolic effects of adding sucrose and aspartame to the diet of subjects with noninsulin dependent diabetes mellitus. *American Journal of Clinical Nutrition* 50: 474–78.

COLEMAN, D. L., ET AL. 1990. Effect of diet on incidences of diabetes in nonobese diabetic mice. *Diabetes* 39: 432–36.

CRANE, M. J. 1994. Sample C. Regression of diabetic neuropathy with total vegetarian (vegan) diet. *Journal of Nutritional Medicine* 4: 431–39.

DAHL-JORGENSEN, K., ET AL. 1991. Relationship between cow's milk consumption and incidences of IDDM in childhood. *Diabetes Care* 14: 1081–83.

DESMET, P. 1997. The role of plant-derived drugs and herbal medicines in healthcare. *Drugs* 54(6): 801–40.

DRAKE, J. A. 1985. *Handbook of Medicinal Herbs*. Boca Raton, Fla.: CRC Press.

FESKENS, E. J. M., et al. 1991. Inverse association between fish intake and risk of glucose intolerance in normal glycemic elderly men and women. *Diabetes Care* 14: 935–41.

GABY, A. R., AND J. V. WRIGHT. 1996. Diabetes. In *Nutritional therapy in medical practice: Reference manual and study guide*, pp. 54–64. Kent, Wash.: Wright/Gaby Seminars.

Goden, G., et al. 1993. Effects of ethanol on carbohydrate metabolism in the elderly. *Diabetes* 42: 28–34.

GREGORY, R. P., AND D. L. DAVIS. 1994. Use of carbohydrate counting for meal planning in type I diabetes. *The Diabetes Educator* 20 (Sept.–Oct.): 514–17.

KLINK, B. 1997. Alternative medicines: Is natural really better? *Drug Topics* (June): 99–103.

LANDIN, K., ET AL. 1992. Guar gum improves insulin sensitivity, blood lipids, blood pressure, and fibrinolysis in healthy men. *American Journal of Clinical Nutrition* 56: 1061–65.

LETTLE, G. J., ET AL. 1987. Glucose and insulin responses to manufactured and whole foods snacks. *American Journal of Clinical Nutrition* 45: 86–91.

LILJEBERG, H., AND I. BJORCH. 1994. Bioavailability of starch in bread products: Postprandial glucose and insulin responses in subjects and in vitro resistant starch content. *European Journal of Clinical Nutrition* 48: 151–63.

LOGHMANI, E., ET AL. 1991. Glycemic response to sucrose-containing mixed meals in diets of children with insulin dependent diabetes mellitus. *Journal of Pediatrics* 119: 531–37.

MERTZ, W. 1992. Chromium: History and nutritional importance. *Biological Trace Element Research* 32: 3–8.

MURRAY, M., AND J. PIZZORNO. 1991. Diabetes mellitus. In *Encyclopedia of Natural Medicines*, pp. 269–85. Rocklin, Calif.: Prima Publishing.

POPP, SNIJDERS, C., ET AL. 1987. Dietary supplementation of omega 3 polyunsaturated fatty acids improves insulin sensitivity in non-insulin dependent diabetes. *Diabetes Research* 4: 141–47.

RUMESSEN, J. J., ET AL. 1990. Fructans of Jerusalem artichokes: Intestinal transport, absorption, fermentation, and influence on blood glucose, insulin, and C-peptide responses in healthy subjects. *American Journal of Clinical Nutrition* 52: 675–81.

SCOTT, F. W. E., ET AL. 1996. Milk and type 1 diabetes. *Diabetes Care* 19: 379–83.

SEELIG, M. S. 1994. Consequences of magnesium deficiency on the enhancement of stress reactions: Preventative and therapeutic implications (a review). *Journal of the American College of Nutrition* 13(5): 429–46.

SHAMBERGER, R. J. 1996. The insulin-like effects of vanadium. *Journal of Advanced Medicine* 9(2): 121–31.

SHANMUGASUNDARAM, E.R.B., ET AL. 1990. Use of Gymnema sylvestre leaf extract in the control of blood glucose in insulin-dependent diabetes mellitus. *Journal of Ethnopharmacology* 30: 281–94.

SNOWDON, D. A., AND R. PHILLIPS. 1985. Does a vegetarian diet reduce the occurrence of diabetes? *American Journal of Public Health* 75: 507–12.

Other books by
Betty Wedman-St. Louis, Ph.D., R. D., L.D.
Quick and Easy Diabetic Menus
Diabetic Desserts
Fast and Fabulous Diabetic Menus
Living with Food Allergies

Index